For appointment call
1-800-317-EYES

Book Excerpts

"I believe Dr. Price's work goes far beyond him, and I hope he realizes this. God is using him to touch lives and work miracles. In essence, Dr. Price is actually giving a new life to each of his patients and there's no way of gauging how far that life reaches and how many other lives will be impacted."

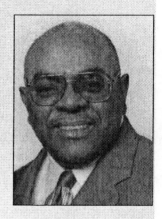

Senior Pastor Clarence Moore

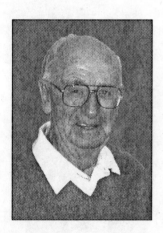

"My life has changed so much since the transplant. It has given my wife and I both a new lease on life. I have been a volunteer in a hospice but had taken a leave because I could no longer drive. Just recently I have been able to get back into it again. And I can play golf now and actually see the ball. ...I am an active, productive member of society again. I can do what I want and I am independent once more."

Robert Higginbotham

"My eye was heavily bandaged and the next day when they took them off, I could see the big "E" on the eye chart! What a thrill! Dr. Price was beaming and happy, of course. It was a miracle really and there was not a dry eye in his office that day. He is so darn good at what he does. He is not someone who would ever give up on you."

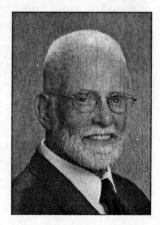

Ed Jagiela

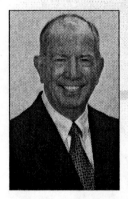

"I think we all have a tendency to take things for granted but I appreciate my blessings now more than ever. I certainly appreciate the fact that some people are devoting their lives to helping others like Dr. Price is doing. He is a humble man, down to earth, but he has this tremendous gift. I truly appreciate the research he's doing. I donate to his Foundation because he is so impressive to me and he is using his gift to benefit mankind... One other thing I want to say is that, unfortunately, sometimes as you get older you are reminded of your age and rather than hearing what can be done to help you, you are discouraged from seeking help. Reject this approach. Find a doctor who wants to help you. You're never too old for good sight."

Donald Wright

"The whole atmosphere in the clinic was so supportive, up-to-date and professional. I learned a lot as I went through the process; it opened new doors of information for me and increased my sense of positive anticipation and eagerness to have the surgery. Finally, after all the doctors I had seen, I had found the right one!"

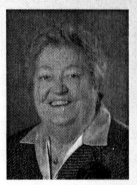

Pat Cowan

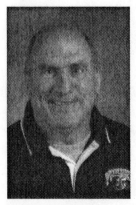

"We have four children (three boys and one girl) and after the surgery, I was able to do things with them that I previously had been reluctant to do. It was exciting from that standpoint. Things like wrestling, camping, swimming together and even being able to get up in the middle of the night with them if they were sick or had a bad dream. I could actually help out and be a full parent without limitations. These are things that most parents take for granted, but I had a new sense of appreciation for them once my vision was restored."

Bob Brock

Celebration of Light

ELAINE VOCI, PH.D.

Cornea Research Foundation of America

Forward by
by Dr. Francis W. Price, Jr.

Bloomington, IN

Milton Keynes, UK

AuthorHouse™
1663 Liberty Drive, Suite 200
Bloomington, IN 47403
www.authorhouse.com
Phone: 1-800-839-8640

AuthorHouse™ UK Ltd.
500 Avebury Boulevard
Central Milton Keynes, MK9 2BE
www.authorhouse.co.uk
Phone: 08001974150

This book is a work of non-fiction. Unless otherwise noted, the author and the publisher make no explicit guarantees as to the accuracy of the information contained in this book and in some cases, names of people and places have been altered to protect their privacy.

First published by AuthorHouse 4/18/2006

ISBN: 1-4259-2725-4 (sc)

Printed in the United States of America
Bloomington, Indiana

This book is printed on acid-free paper.

Parable of the Talents

Matthew 25:14

" Stay alert for you do not know the day or the hour. For it is just like a man about to go on a journey who called his servants and entrusted his possessions to them. To one he gave five talents, to another, two and to a third, one, each according to his ability. He went on the journey and was gone a long time. Upon his return, the first servant had traded the talents to make five more; the second had done the same and made two more; but the third had buried the one talent in the ground and returned it with no gain. The man was pleased with the first two servants and invited them to join into his joy, but the third he cast out. For everyone who has, more will be given and he will have abundance. Whoever does not have, even what he has will be taken from him."

This is one of my favorite Bible passages. It reminds me that being a good servant involves choosing to use the talents loaned to us by God for His Higher Purposes, taking risks in order to grow and advance them, while being a good steward over the talents as long as they are in our care.

It requires surrendering to His will over and over, trusting His will, and living for others, not just ourselves. I hope that my life's work will be a living demonstration of these beliefs and values, and I am grateful to each of the people in this book whose lives deepen my faith.

Francis W. Price, Jr. M.D.

Contents

Myopia

Fuchs' Dystrophy

Laser Refractive Surgery

Other Conditions

Preface

Writing this book has been the proverbial "labor of love" for me. Each patient that I met has been such a gift to me personally as they related their journeys and I got to know them. Their courage, their dogged determination, and their faith uplift me.

The book title, *Celebration of Light,* speaks to the inspiration that you will find in the patients' stories, as well as the education you will gain from reading Dr. Price's comments in the Foreward.

All proceeds of the book, including royalties, go to the Foundation to support its life-changing work. We are indebted to Tom Britt and AuthorHouse for publishing our book at no charge as a charitable donation to the Foundation. We appreciate Jim Cota, President and Creative Director of Rare Bird for the beautiful cover art created by his amazing graphic artist, Troy Chandler, as an in-kind donation to the Foundation. Thank you!

Chapters

The chapters are based on taped interview sessions conducted with each person and, in a few cases, with their spouses who attended the interviews. Most interviews were done on the telephone, although in some cases, I drove to the person's home or met them after they finished an appointment with Dr. Price in Indianapolis. In addition to taping their stories,

I also relied on written notes that I took during interviews to then transcribe the chapters in each person's own words, with some editing of content to allow for a smooth, logical sequencing of their story.

Taking this approach, my goal is that readers will feel as if they having a private, informal conversation with each speaker.

How This Book Is Organized

(A) The Table of Contents groups chapters by eye condition, then by the name of the individual and by chapter title.

(B) The Glossary in the back of the book contains descriptions of various eye terms you will encounter in the stories and others that relate to common surgeries and procedures available in Dr.Price's modern ophthalmology practice.

(C) A description of the Foundation can be found at the end of the book including the history of its inception in 1988, and how to donate.

Elaine Voci, Ph.D.

Introduction

by Elaine Voci, Ph.D.

Our eyes are sacred. We understand that we have been given one pair, most of us, from birth and they have to last us a lifetime. When we think of losing our sight, it strikes fear in our hearts. We quickly imagine all that we would miss: the faces of our loved ones, the many beautiful sunrises and sunsets we have been inspired by, and the independent lifestyle we have taken for granted. For most of us, being sighted is central to the experience of being totally, fully human.

When disease or disabling conditions threaten our sight, or that of a loved one, it is difficult at first to muster the clarity of mind to know what to do. In this age of machines, many of us go to the World Wide Web and begin researching everything we can get our hands on. We access medical information that just a decade ago was unavailable to all but the medical professional. It brings comfort and knowledge, but can also add confusion and even misinformation. If only we could find and talk to someone else who has faced the same challenges, we may think to ourselves.

And that is the first reason why this book was written.

The stories in *Celebration of Light are* a generous gift of the human spirit from a group of individuals who faced vision challenges, and in some cases, the loss of sight. Some of them struggled for years just to find out what was wrong with their eyes. As children, many endured the painful experience of being made to feel different, a stigma that continues today for the visually impaired. Each of them dealt with their circumstances through various coping strategies, such as humor, risk-taking, a tireless quest for information, and the loving support of friends and family.

Knowledge is power. Understanding the condition we face, what our options are and what to expect from treatment instills strength, courage and hope in us. We move from the darkness of fearful imaginings to the light of informed choices.

That is the second reason why this book was written.

Dr. Francis Price, Jr., helped these patients make wise choices about their vision. An internationally recognized ophthalmic surgeon, he has been named one of the top physicians in the country for corneal disease and transplantation by THE BEST DOCTORS IN AMERICA and, in 2005, Ophthalmologist of the Year by the Indiana Academy of Ophthalmology. A diligent and prolific researcher, he has published more than 80 study articles in peer-reviewed journals and served as Principal Investigator in 62 clinical research studies. His observations in the Foreward provide insight into some of the common corneal conditions, including Fuchs' Dystrophy and keratoconus, as well as some unusual ones like aniridia.

The individuals whose stories are featured in *Celebration of Light* provide practical and spiritual advice to readers:
- Do your homework
- Seek support from other people
- Evaluate medical resources
- Find the best physicians
- Continue to have faith in the future
- Be grateful for each and every day for it is a blessing

That is the third reason why this book was written.

All proceeds from this book go to the Cornea Research Foundation of America which was started in 1988 by Dr. Price. He was prompted by the desire to do something no one else was doing at the time: to keep track of the outcomes of corneal transplants. Within ten years, the Foundation amassed the largest cornea transplant database in the Western Hemisphere that continues to help surgeons enhance long-term graft survival. Today, the Foundation conducts at least 12 annual studies that contribute to advances in refractive surgery, cataract surgery, treatment of presbyopia (old eyes) and treatments for iris problems. Three years ago, Marianne Price, Ph.D., joined her husband of thirty years as Director of Research and Education. Together they are pioneering new surgical techniques, promising new devices and medications for his patients, as well as providing education for surgeons around the world.

Celebration of Light is, thus, a fund-raiser for the Foundation and that is the final reason why this book was written. We hope you will partner with us and share knowledge of this book widely with as many family and friends as you are able. We hope they will visit our website and attend our free bi-annual Open Houses and ask to be put on our mailing list to receive free copies of our quarterly newsletter, the Visionary. Together we can help bring a healing light of hope and discoveries to truly celebrate the precious gift of sight.

Foreward

by Dr. Francis W. Price, Jr.

Is anyone ever too old for a corneal transplant? We might as well ask, "Does anyone ever reach the point where they are too old to see?" I don't think so. Fifty years ago, it was common to expect people to naturally become blind, deaf and immobile as they aged. Today we expect elders to be able to continue to enjoy excellent vision, hearing and mobility. Our standards and definition of aging have dramatically altered. The choice is really between darkness and light. And since vision is key to human communication and understanding, no one is ever too old to improve his or her sight. As you will discover, this book is a superb affirmation of that belief.

Elaine has done a wonderful job of capturing the feelings and concerns of a variety of patients I have been fortunate enough to meet and help with their vision problems. A common thread you will find in their stories is that many had given up hope as they struggled to carry out normal daily activities with their conditions. They had either been told there was nothing that could be done, or that the proposed treatments were undesirable or insufficiently tested. I reject such "advice" and I think it is important not to give up hope and, instead, to continually find better ways to do things.

Advances only occur when we push the envelope, or take risks to try something new. I encourage my staff to do this, and I adhere to that principle myself in continually trying to find better ways to treat or fix problems our patients have with vision challenges. We should never accept status quo as the best we can do.

People frequently ask me if there will be better treatments for their problems in the future, compared to what I can offer now. I have a standard response: "I certainly hope so." Wouldn't it be sad if we could not expect continual improvements to emerge? Life is full of change and our knowledge and techniques, aided by technology, constantly provide us with new information, insights and ideas that have practical applications. The field of ophthalmology does not exist in a vacuum; it is part of the great wheel of human progress that keeps turning. We don't know when new advances might take place; it could be tomorrow or it could be in the next millennium. But in the meantime, everyone should be encouraged to seek the latest treatments and procedures available.

There are several key points I want to make as you begin reading *Celebration of Light:*

- The stories in this book are about people who have experienced positive life changing results from surgery. I want to caution you that not all surgery has a happy ending; complications can and do occur. Still, most people do benefit greatly from these remarkable procedures.

- Most of the conditions described include those that are secondary to injury, infection or heredity and are easily recognized, such as cataracts, corneal scars or corneal distortions.

- Other conditions were not considered diseases or abnormalities appropriate for surgery when I began treating them. These were the eyes with nearsightedness, or myopia to use the technical term. When I started treating patients with myopia, many doctors at the time thought it was a mistake because such eyes were regarded as "normal." As you read the stories of myopia please keep that historical footnote in mind. Fortunately, as technology advanced, we were able to make changes and get very good results. Today, twenty years later, it is widely accepted that treating myopia is a good thing and can make a huge difference in a patient's quality of life.

A Common Question

Our Foundation is named the Cornea Research Foundation of America. So, you might ask, "Why do you treat conditions that don't seem to be corneal?" The answer is simple: when treating corneal conditions, we often end up treating related and complex problems with the anterior, or front, part of the eye. That is why we have to carry out complicated surgical reconstruction of the eye after certain types of injuries. For example, aniridia is a disease in which the iris is missing either due to heredity or injury. It can affect the cornea. In fact, in the hereditary type of aniridia, scarring, diminished retinal function, reduced vision and glaucoma often go hand in hand with scarring of the cornea.

Another hereditary disease that impacts the cornea is Fuchs' Dystrophy. As it progresses, little bumps, or guttata, form on the inner surface of the cornea. These lead to the distortion of light going through the cornea and eventually reduce vision and increase glare. Ultimately, most people with Fuchs' Dystrophy develop painful bulli, or blisters, on the eye. It has been gratifying to be able to help develop a more successful way of treating this challenging condition and increase the quality of life for so many.

Many of you will recognize another condition described in the book known as keratoconus. This condition weakens the cornea and causes the eye to bulge out like a weak spot on a bicycle tire. Instead of the usual round shape, the eye becomes oval like a football. Transplants have worked well for this condition for many years, but there really needs to be new and improved treatment procedures found and increased efforts made toward prevention. Our Foundation is making this one of our research goals in the next decade. We will be working hard to innovate new treatments and uncover the causes of this disabling condition. Hopefully, many of you will feel the desire to join us on this mission by donating your time, talent and financial support to the Foundation.

In Closing

It is my intention that this book will live up to its title, and bring a sense of hope and renewal to our readers. When Elaine proposed the concept to me almost a year ago, I was intrigued. I knew I would personally learn from patients' stories told in their own words and I knew they would be able to touch the lives of many. What better bridge can there be for those who are searching for information and inspiration, than to hear from peers who, suffering the same conditions, took the necessary risks to move forward with hope, faith and courage?

To each of the people in this book who were willing to share their personal experiences, I celebrate you! It is a joy and a privilege to have been of help and I admire your tenacity, your sense of humor and your inspiring outlook on life. I am proud of each of you for reaching out to assist those you may never meet. Bless you.

To those who have found their way to this book and will use it as a resource and a decision-making tool, I also celebrate you! In your heart lies a knowing self, a Higher Self, and it has led you to this moment and to this group of loving, kind individuals whose stories await within. Enjoy them, savor their wise recommendations, and whatever you choose to do about your vision challenges, know that you are not alone.

To my clinical staff, and to Dr. Kathy Kelley and Dr. Faye Peters, I want you to know how proud I am of you as I read these stories and the repeated complements about how well you have cared for our patients. You surely can see for yourself the impact you are having. You are an amazing group of people and I am deeply grateful that you continually strive to deliver your best, each and every day. Thank you for being such a wonderful team!

To my wife, Marianne, thank you for being my best friend, my best colleague and my best co-author on so many clinical research papers. I am indebted to you more than I can put into words and you are my inspiration.

To my parents, Francis and Marion, I appreciate everything you have done to provide a solid foundation upon which to build my life's work. You are a remarkable pair and much loved by all of us in our family. I hope you will enjoy reading these stories and feel a part of the journey, for it all began with you.

To my four children, Patrick, Mark, Diane and David, my daughter-in-law Sara and my grandchildren, Miguel and Marianna, I hope this book will be a lasting legacy of love for you to carry into the future.

Finally, to my Board of Directors, may this book bring you inspiration and renewed commitment to our mission. Our work together is a continual source of revitalization to me and I appreciate all that you do to help us successfully achieve our goals with grace and wisdom.

Myopia

"Thank You Very Much!"

Bob Brock is a high school principal with an outgoing personality and his story is filled with achievements on the athletic field as well as in the game of life. Reflective at times, humorous at others, Bob's insights during his interview show how he has been "seasoned" by life's challenges and heartened by its victories. His sense of risk-taking and adventure were both in play when he became part of an Artisan lens study and met two doctors who would change his life for the better.

Dr. Kelley and I are close; she is a neat gal and the one who really helped me through this thing. Occasionally she refers people to me who are considering eye surgery. I talk to them and am honest with them regarding the pros and cons of the procedure I had which is called an Artisan lens.* It makes me feel good to help others and so I am glad to be part of this book.

My Background

My vision problems most likely began at birth but it wasn't until I was four years old that my parents noticed how I had to sit really close to the TV in order to watch programs. They took me for an eye exam and were told that I needed glasses to correct extreme myopia and stigmatism. I started wearing glasses - and breaking them regularly - because I played all kinds of sports and was always wrestling with my siblings and kids in the neighborhood. Luckily, my Dad was the kind of guy who kept his soldering gun out with the wire and drill ever handy so he could keep my glasses together.   At one point my parents even invested in a pair of big heavy duty athletic glasses complete with a nose pad and aluminum that you could run over with a car. Those things were pretty indestructible, even for a kid like me.

My folks were wonderfully supportive of my athletic events and came to everything I ever did. My desire to play was just so strong. My Dad played football for the Chicago Bears and the Chicago Cardinals. He also graduated from the University of Kentucky. Down deep in his heart, as a father, he wanted me to be safe, but he knew how much football meant to me because it meant a lot to him. We had been going to games up at Wrigley Field forever and he enjoyed taking me. He just knew that I loved the game and when he saw that look in my eyes, he knew I had to play.

I was in the eighth grade when I was told I could not play because of my glasses, and I remember I welled up when I heard those words. Being an athlete was everything to me, right or wrong, and my mission became finding a doctor who would permit me to play, and we finally did. My retina had really been stretched because of my myopia. One of the things my Dad told me back then was to build up my neck and shoulders to absorb any blows in order to protect my head. I followed his advice and didn't have any serious injuries.

I was a linebacker and played for Crown Pointe High School. In addition, I played baseball, basketball and wrestling. All of these sports were hard to play with glasses on so, when they came out with hard contact lenses, I thought it was great. Of course, the downside was that I kept losing them all the time. We went through a lot of them! It became obvious that both glasses and contact lenses each had drawbacks, so I opted to wear glasses until my sophomore year in high school. I tried wearing contacts again for a year and then resigned myself to glasses which I wore through college at Butler University where I successfully played football and, later, for the Cleveland Browns professional team.

Finding Dr. Price and Dr. Kathy Kelley

I was wearing glasses when I first heard Dr. Price's name and the word LASIK. I was working out at a health club and the guy I worked out with had just had LASIK done. As bad as my vision was, his had been worse. It made a huge difference in his life and he could see better than 20/20 afterwards. Dr. Price had performed the laser surgery and that's how I got his name. I called for an appointment soon after and went to see him in Indianapolis.

The first thing Dr. Price told me was that I had to wear "Coke bottle" glasses for three weeks before surgery to let my eyes "round out" again. Truthfully, I was blind most of those three weeks because I had a little too much vanity and didn't want to anyone to see me in those things.

I went back in three weeks and they said I couldn't have the procedure. My eyesight was so bad and my eyeball was too out of round which meant they would have to shave too much off. I was bummed and I regretted that they hadn't told me that was a possibility in the first place. Then Dr. Kelley came in and talked to me. That was the first time I met her.

She told me about a new program, the "Artisan claw" lens, which was not federally approved yet and asked me to consider it in order to improve my vision. It was a device that would be attached to my iris with tiny hooks, hence the term "claw." Dr. Price was the Principal Investigator and she was the Clinical Research Coordinator for the project. I did not want to have my eyes slit and something put in them. I was put off by the whole idea. There were so many things about it that were experimental. By then it was phase three of a long-term study and I would be a guinea pig. Insurance wouldn't cover it and if something went wrong, it would be serious.

I put my contacts back in and went home to think it over. Dr. Price called that night and talked to me in greater detail about the procedure. He sent me some things to read and then Dr. Kelley talked to me again, too. For some reason those two people, Dr. Kelley and Dr. Price, instilled in me a great deal of confidence in their skills. I didn't feel like I was a lab animal and I sensed that they sincerely cared about my vision and me. They were convinced that I would be helped by the procedure.

We were dealing with something that was a bit unknown since it was still being tested. I did some Internet research to learn more but I was still hesitant. I was afraid that someday I might not be able to wear contacts anymore and I would have to go back to wearing those awful glasses. My worst fear was that I would become so limited that I would lose my independence.

I had faith in both doctors about being part of the study and accepting the procedure. I did my homework and talked to a couple of other people who were already in the study. I also talked it over with my wife and my mother and they were in agreement that I should "give it a shot!" I'm not so conservative that I won't try something new, and that was part of my decision-making process, too.

I also had a good first impression of Dr. Price; he was calm and professional and I weighed that in my decision. He wasn't in it for the money, and I really felt he was in it for me. He was able to offer me something that would be long-lasting that I would feel good about. Let's face it: I had severe myopia and it couldn't get much worse. The condition had kept me out of the service, for example, so it was kind of a miracle that I wasn't walking with a cane! I bucked the idea a bit at first; I wasn't sure about it. Neither Dr. Price nor Dr. Kelley tried to sell me on being in the study but they were so sincere and genuinely concerned about me that they won me over. I remember at one point, Dr. Price said, "Hey, let's go for it." And so we did.

My Surgery

The day of the surgery I woke up feeling a little nervous, but excited. I arrived at the facility and went to the surgical area. When it was my turn, I was draped and kept awake the whole time, able to talk to the doctors as they operated. They kept a good conversation going with me, step by step, and it was very reassuring. They used numbing drops for the eye and I was comfortable. I did not have any pain. No adverse affects at all. They kept putting drops in my eye as they worked and they explained what they were doing the whole time.

I couldn't feel anything; for example, when they told me they needed to move the lens, I could feel a tug but nothing else. Dr. Price and I even cracked a few jokes and laughed together. I did not feel a great deal of anxiety even while the surgery was underway. It was not traumatic.

After it was finished, I wore a patch on that eye for a day or so, and had a friend drive me back and forth to the clinic. I rested at home and then came back to the clinic for periodic checkups. For the first week, I had to put an ointment in my eye. It all went so smoothly. My vision was 20/35 and it's still that today! I have been able to pass the vision test to drive and I only wear glasses to read.

It was hard for me to believe that I could have such clear vision without a contact lens. I had prepared myself so well and believed in Dr. Price so much, I think I expected to see clearly. So when it actually happened, it was just the way he and I both thought it would turn out. It was one of those experiences where you just wanted to say, "Thank you very much!"

Of course, once that first eye went so well, I was eager to have the second eye done. It was quite a summer for me; I had the first eye done at the start of the summer and three months later, I had the second procedure.

How Life Changed

My wife Patsy and I had been a camping couple and people that didn't know us would see us holding hands walking up to the restrooms together, for example, or I would have my hand on her shoulders. People would think we were such a close couple. What they didn't know was that I couldn't see and she was like my Seeing Eye guide. Achieving improved vision liberated my wife, too, from my being so dependent on her when I didn't have my glasses or contacts in.

Little things like being able to see the clock in the morning and not having to worry if I fell asleep in front of the TV that I had to remember to take my lenses out, stuff like that really made a difference in the quality of life. Life itself had improved not just my vision.

We have four children (three boys and one girl) and after the surgery, I was able to do things with them that I previously had been reluctant to do. It was exciting from that standpoint. Things like wrestling, camping, swimming together and even being able to get up in the middle of the night with them if they were sick or had a bad dream. I could actually help out and be a full parent without limitations. These are things that most parents take for granted, but I had a new sense of appreciation for them once my vision was restored.

There is a relationship between football and choosing to have this procedure. Athletics and football teaches you so many lessons in life. It develops your personality and your inner resilience; you learn how to lose and how to win. It gives you confidence in yourself. That background enabled me to approach the surgical procedure with confidence in a practical mindset and myself. If something bad happened and my eyes did not improve, I would not collapse or lose my faith. We would have just taken the lens out and I would not have been any worse off.

Life Lessons

God has been awful good to me in my life. If you met me in person, you would see that I walk with a limp. That is because I was a quadriplegic and on a respirator for two years. I was in Methodist Hospital in 1988 for four months being treated for Guillain-Barre Syndrome (a disorder in which the body's immune system attacks part of the peripheral nervous system). It happened when I had knee surgery to treat an old football injury, and my antibodies attacked my nervous system. The doctors did not know if I would ever walk again.

I had a lot of doctors who talked to me during that period of my life and I learned to have faith, more faith than I ever had. It wasn't like I found God because I had always believed in Him, but it deepened my faith. I always felt that you played the hand that was dealt, and this was another opportunity to practice that belief. Looking back, I feel it made me a better person.

I was so competitive that it actually helped me heal. If I walked two feet one day, I wanted to walk three the next time. It drove me quite a bit. I had my ups and downs, of course, and cried like a little girl some days, but then I'd fight like mad the next.

My legs are not really strong any longer but I have learned to adapt. I can't run upstairs anymore, but I still workout and I ride a stationary bike. I'm not the same athlete in that it's slowed me down a little which has only made me more appreciative of my family and friends. I realize how important they are and that's been one of the biggest benefits. You know, we all go through life and paddle along but then something like that happens and we see things very differently. I am sure I drew strength from this life experience as I faced the decisions about being part of a study and having surgery on my eyes.

Looking back, I would absolutely do it again. It comes down to the quality of life you want to have. Today, this lens has been approved so now there is a high rate of successful outcomes. You can feel confidence in it. But you should still ask every question you can think of, and do research to find out as much as you can. I have spoken to many people and each person just has to make them- selves feel comfortable with the procedure. If they want an improved quality of life, I encourage them to have the surgery because I definitely believe it will be worthwhile.

If anyone reading this would like to talk to me personally, please tell him or her to contact me. I can come and visit them and would be happy to do that. It's so important and I was helped so much by this procedure that I am glad to take the time to help someone else.

Note: The Artisan® lens study conducted at the Foundation contributed to FDA approval of this device. The purpose of the study was to evaluate whether placing a lens in the eye could safely correct high levels of near-sightedness. It was determined to be safe and effective. In North America, the lens is known as the Verisyse® lens and is available to other patients who might benefit from it.

Myopia

"An IMAX World"

Ken Swedo is an engineer working in military service to his country. He employs the same accuracy and precision in telling his story as he does to maintaining F/A-18 jet fighter planes. One of Dr. Price's first patients, Ken recalls those early days when the office was small, and the receptionist was the surgeon's mother. Since then, the practice has grown substantially and Ken has become a faithful supporter of the Foundation that Dr. Price began in 1988. Ken's story illustrates the life-changing power that is possible when a skilled surgeon, an innovative method and a patient's positive attitude are combined.

I was born in Chicago and living there when I became severely and suddenly myopic. I was in the third grade at the time. I started wearing thick glasses and became consistently more near-sighted with each passing year. My visual deterioration finally leveled off in high school. By then I was wearing heavy glasses which were really unattractive. I also had light-sensitive eyes and so I had to wear photochromatic, darkening lenses. These glasses were not made in any fashionable styles, either, so that didn't help my general appearance any. Sports were difficult, and so I gravitated toward Chess and became a good player. I was more comfortable with things I could get my arms around than with physical outdoor activities taking place fifty yards down a field.

With my condition, images were always distorted. I naturally saw things smaller. When I got up in the morning, I had to grab the clock and put it in front of my face, for example, in order to see the time.

When I got into college, I started wearing soft contact lenses. I had some additional problems because with my strong prescription, not all contacts were made in the strength I needed. I also have tight eyelids, so the contacts would actually irritate my eyes because the lenses would drift up in the eyelid. The more irritation, the more they grabbed and a snowball effect would kick in. I also had a bad experience with a new type of wafer-thin lens, advertised as 24-hour lenses that you never took out. They tended to really dry my eyes out and it felt like sandpaper in my eyes each morning. To make a long story short, after six months, I just could not wear them anymore and went back to wearing glasses.

A New Young Doctor and
A Promising New Procedure

I first met Dr. Price through stories about him in the newspaper, on radio and TV. I remember quite vividly how the newspaper and TV stories made me feel intrigued and excited. Back then, it was not like today when everyone does laser surgery and it's ho-hum. At that time, he was the only one performing a groundbreaking surgical procedure called myopic keratomileusis. This is a method of reshaping the corneal surface to change its optical power to correct extreme refractive errors, especially near-sightedness like I had. A disc of the cornea is shaved off, quickly frozen, lathe-ground and then returned to its original position. The procedure was first developed in the 1960's by a Colombian doctor, I believe, and then brought to Indy by Dr. Price. It was cutting edge!

Dr. Price was definitely someone I wanted to meet and talk to about this new procedure. The surgery sounded like an answer to my dreams that could correct my vision. The highest expectation I hoped for was that I would be able to get out of thick glasses and into thin ones. I thought if I could come out of the operation with 20/40 vision, I would be thrilled.

When I called Dr. Price's office for an informational meeting, I met with a man named Rick Kadel in a very small office. (I also got to meet Dr. Price's mother, Marian, because she was the receptionist.) Rick was a senior assistant to the doctor and a fantastic teacher, very knowledgeable. He really helped answer my questions - and I had a lot of them. In fact, later on Rick would say that I had more questions than all of the other patients combined!

We discussed the surgical risks, the possibility of failure, the expenses; he was very honest and never put any pressure on me to make a decision. Now keep in mind that this was when Dr. Price was a young doctor just starting to build his practice. There was a lot of competition in the city and it would have been easy, and understandable, for Rick to push me into having the surgery. Instead, he remained caring, attentive and respectful of my decision-making process. I took my time and weighed the information carefully.

When I subsequently met with Dr. Price, I found him to have an extremely good manner. He was candid, described the procedure in detail and patiently answered my questions. In fact, he was as detail-oriented as I was and that was great. I am an engineer and technical skills matter as much as knowledge in my field. Dr. Price had this quiet self-confidence about him, and he had a great track record of successful procedures. He told me that a laser method had already been envisioned to bring about the same results, but he was not sure when it would be introduced or how good the results would be. I spoke with several of his patients who had already had the procedure and they gave me candid feedback that was very useful. After processing all the information I had learned, I decided to go ahead with it.

The Surgery

Before the procedure was done I took a battery of tests that measured the eye from a number of angles to ensure optimal results. Dr. Price was very thorough. The surgery was performed on one eye at a time; each procedure took four to six months to really heal. In my case, we opted to do the left eye, my worst eye, first.

I was put under while he put a shot behind my eye to immobilize it and to deaden it so that it wouldn't move. He then put a ring on the eye to hold it in place. He took a special surgical blade and cut across the corneal surface to "flatten" the surface. Then he took the part he had cut off, flash froze it, and put it on a cryolathe, a computer-controlled machine, to re-cut the piece and remove tissue on each side. Then it was unfrozen and sutured back onto the eye. It's pretty unbelievable how intricate and perfect the sutures were. I could have stared at them for hours if I had been given access to a photo of them. They were in a star pattern throughout the eye and it was really an incredible image.

My first surgery was a perfect surgery, a "bulls eye" result. It took 2 hours to prepare for surgery, and then one hour for the actual procedure and another 1.5 hours to recover and be sent home with a patch and a small metal shield to protect the eye. The next day, I came in for an exam followed by weekly exams and then, gradually, monthly visits. During this time, I had an antibiotic cream to apply to prevent infection from developing, and I had to sleep upright. Soon after surgery, I was able to resume normal activities including driving and, eventually, I had the patch removed but kept the metal guard on at night while sleeping.

The improvement was gradual over 4-5 months time, but my vision was improved to 20/15! It far exceeded my expectations. I could see better than I ever could before with either glasses or contact lenses! One unexpected outcome was that everything I could now see so clearly seemed huge. Even my eyes themselves felt huge to me, like watermelons. It felt like I was seeing things in a giant IMAX world. It took me awhile to get adjusted to the sensation.

Dr. Price was patient and did not hurry to do the other eye. He wanted to be sure there were no complications so we waited about 9 months. The only side effect I experienced, besides the sense of having huge eyes, was a moderate amount of haze and afterglow in my night vision. I could see a kind of halo around headlights or streetlights, but eventually this disappeared.

We repeated the operation on my other eye and, while the results were very good, they were not perfect, as my first one had been. I became a little less farsighted with astigmatism and I have since had some regression with my first eye, so now I am nearsighted. But it worked out fine. In fact, sometimes this result is intentionally pursued in order to help patients have balanced vision. I use the right eye for distance and my left eye for close-ups and I won't have to wear bifocals or reading glasses when I get older.

How Life Has Changed

I see more clearly now and without the thick, heavy, cumbersome glasses I had to wear before. I am not a vain person, but it's nice to be like other people. My interests and my personality have gradually moved outward and I have pursued new outdoor activities and have reached out to more people. I feel like I have a better connectivity with the outside world and in that sense, my world has expanded. I am grateful for that.

As an engineer, I respect the new techniques that modern medicine and sciences are constantly developing that add to our quality of life. We have to be open to these discoveries and to doctors who are doing cutting edge work. It would be so much easier for a doctor, once they have that medical degree, to just go with the flow and not do what is more difficult or challenging. We are very lucky that people like Dr. Price are around who are willing to take the lead. There is a heck of a lot of others, I am sure, who stand on his shoulders for the research he's done since 1988. I know he and his wife, Marianne Price, Ph.D., both have good strong scientific backgrounds and they make sure that what they do is repeatable, measurable and can be used to help people. All progress is usually a succession of small steps and as long as you make each of these steps strong, there will be advances.

Advice to Readers

From my personal standpoint, I think you should be aware that obstacles can be overcome by radical change. Be open to that.

Choose your surgeon very carefully. Check their credentials, and experience and the equipment that they use. It might be tough for laymen to do, but you really have to conduct your own research.

Carefully weigh the risks and benefits. Check out the options you have during surgery and afterwards. Ask questions. Develop a plan for all contingencies. Be prepared for everything. Knowledge takes away the unknown and the fear of the unknown.

If you decide to go ahead, remember that a positive attitude is very important to deal with the procedure. A positive attitude can definitely influence the result according to the anecdotal evidence I have read. I draw my own strength and courage from maintaining a positive attitude and accepting the support of my family and friends, and the doctor and his staff. I also draw strength from knowledge and understanding.

Be patient after the surgery. There is a period of fluctuation in the vision and the final result may not be known for some time. It's not like Laser surgery where you have a rapid result.

Avoid unrealistic expectations. Be positive but realize that nothing is ever promised; everything you will achieve is a bonus. You wouldn't go into the operation unless you had positive expectations, but don't expect perfection. Some things are unavoidable, short and long-term, and you just have to face them.

In closing, I would like to extend my thanks to Dr. Price and to Robin, his assistant, and his staff in the surgery center, for what they did for me back in the mid-eighties and for the contributions Dr. Price is making to the field of ophthalmology. I think some people are researchers and others are practitioners. Dr. Price is a hybrid; he is both! His perspective is unique. And the synergy is wonderful; his patients benefit from the research and sometimes they directly participate in it.

Vision is a great gift and most people take it for granted. If you have ever been threatened with the loss of your vision, that casual attitude changes in a hurry. You quickly appreciate the work being done by people like Dr. Price and the Foundation to help patients that they are in contact with, as well as many others. His work touches other doctors who read his research and then they use it to advance their own work. Eventually, it helps untold patients, people who may never meet Dr. Price or even know his name.

I am just really glad he has the energy to do it all. I could not. At the end of the day, I am done! He's working a lot of hours, I know, and he works hard so I appreciate all of his achievements. For one person, he has accomplished a lot already and that is an inspiring message for the rest of us.

Myopia

"Coke Bottle Glasses"

Laurie Wolcott is a good historian who methodically describes life events in candid detail without embellishment. She is also a risk-taker, able to generate courage and faith when it is needed. Having been born visually challenged, she underwent a corrective procedure as an adult that enables her to now see clearly without the thick glasses that accompanied her earlier life. This clarity of vision is more than physical; it is also spiritual and metaphorical in that Laurie gauges what is truly significant through a practiced and grateful discernment. Her career change from librarian to minister is almost complete. It is a loving demonstration of her deep, abiding faith in God's wisdom.

I don't remember my first vision challenge because it happened so early in my life. The family story is this: I was very young and learning to roll a ball when an uncle of mine noticed that I couldn't locate the ball after it had stopped rolling. I think that was the first inkling my parents had that something was wrong with my eyes. I was fitted for my first pair of thick glasses when I was just three years old. Then I was watched very carefully for the first five to ten years by my doctors to be sure that I was not going to be blind. I've been told since that I am at great risk for retinal separation.

I haven't seen well all of my life due to a condition termed "severe myopia" that my son has inherited. It presented many struggles when I was a young child. For example, I recall

17

being on a baseball field in elementary school and the physical education teacher yelling at me, "What's the matter? Are you afraid of the ball?" Since I have gotten older, I have realized that yes, I *was* afraid of the ball because I couldn't see it coming until it was right on top of me.

Apart from the physical challenges, I was also challenged academically by myopia. I always did well in school but I could not see the board when I was a kid, and my teachers were not accustomed to working with a child with vision issues. I was an extremely shy child, and I felt different than the other kids. Overall, I functioned pretty well socially, but the "Coke bottle" glasses I wore by the time I got into high school were pretty ugly.

I never considered how big an issue my vision was until I became an adult. In raising my son, it has been amazingly helpful to actually know, from personal experience, what he is going through at various stages. I can explain things to my husband and to my son's teachers. My son wears contacts, which I was unable to do until I was a senior in high school. But his teachers still need to be reminded of his challenges because even with contacts, he cannot see the board. If someone is showing transparencies, for example, he is unable to see them. I believe that people like the two of us simply have to work harder than others do.

I think many of us don't often realize how much of a social thing our vision is; for example, you can't recognize people if you are working hard to focus elsewhere. If someone passes by you when you are focused on something else, your visual field is limited and you simply don't see him or her. As I have gotten older and been in situations where recognition of others matters a lot, I have had to make it a point to tell my congregations, "Trip me, hit me, but please recognize that I am not ignoring you; I just don't see you."

Finding Help

Dr. David Landow is an optometrist in town and he has made a tremendous difference in my life by being willing to work with my contacts. I had a hard time finding a doctor willing to do that. When he told me about the Verisyse lens implant surgery that had been approved, he didn't just tell me about it, he picked up the phone and spoke with Dr. Kathy Kelley in Dr. Price's office. She made an immediate adjustment in her schedule and saw me that same day for a consultation. It was so helpful to get cooperation and attention like that from both of them.

I learned that the FDA approved the first implantable "Verisyse" lens for nearsightedness in the late 90's, giving people with extremely poor eyesight like me a new way to see the world. The lens is attached to the iris, the colored part of the eye, and is an alternative to glasses, contact lenses and LASIK surgery. Dr. Price participated in the approval study and has implanted over 150 of these lenses since 1998.

When I met with Dr. Kelley, she had the office run preliminary tests to determine if I was a candidate for surgery in both eyes. By the time I left her office that day, I knew that I was a good candidate for it, and I also learned, unfortunately, that it would not be covered by my insurance.

Looking back on that February afternoon as I left the office, I felt a little stunned. I did not have time to think about it and absorb all of the information I had been given, but I was grateful and hopeful that this could work and make a significant difference in my life. I was concerned about getting the financing together but my mother was such a blessing. I think it meant as much to her as it did to me; she cried tears of joy when I first told her about it, and she immediately offered to pay for the surgery.

I formed some basic "first impressions" of everyone in the office that day. I thought they were a wonderful and helpful group. Later, when I met Dr. Price, he was both kind and businesslike. Surgery is his specialty and he was knowledgeable to talk to about the procedure. Dr. Kelley was so good, too, because she always took time to answer my questions and she gave me time to think.

The First Surgery

We did the left eye first to be sure it was going to work out and because I was a bit nervous about having surgery on my right eye, my "good" eye. I wouldn't have done it at all if I hadn't trusted the office and I was comforted by the fact that Dr. Price had been doing the procedure for eight years. The fact that it had been the subject of a formal clinical study was impressive and reassuring to me.

The procedure was pretty straightforward. I was given a set of instructions ahead of time. I arrived at the office on the appointed day and filled out the necessary paperwork. I brought my friend, Angie, who is a nurse and she was a calming presence. I got undressed and put on surgical scrubs and was given an IV. Everything ran smoothly and the environment felt calm the whole time I was there.

I had never been wheeled on a gurney anywhere and it provided an unusual perspective of the world as I lay flat and looked up and around my environment. The anesthesiologist came in and she was extraordinarily kind. I was given enough medication in the eye itself and in the IV not to feel any pain and to be able to relax. A drape was laid over my face with a cutout for the eye being operated on and a device was used to keep the eye open. The hardest part for me was to keep my left eye still because I didn't have much control over it. I had to be constantly reminded to keep it as still as I could.

At one point all I could see was darkness and then very quickly I could see the light again so then I knew that things were going as planned. The surgical team was good about explaining what was happening and that was helpful. Dr.

Price talked to me during surgery and I can recall that he kept cautioning me about keeping my left eye still.

When it was finished, I went back to the recovery room. I couldn't have had nicer treatment from nicer people. They had told me it would take about 30 minutes for the surgery itself. I don't recall how long it took but I think we were on target. My friend took me home and that night I attended a seminary class with her. I stayed only for about half of the class because I wasn't supposed to be there at all, following doctor's orders. I felt very little discomfort after the surgery although I was tired that night.

The next day, I had an exam at Dr. Price's office and everything looked fine. He had implanted the lens and corrected my astigmatism to some degree. At that point, I was not wearing correction glasses and on the way to breakfast, I actually read a street sign out loud and my friend was amazed. There had been an immediate improvement in my vision!

The recovery period was two months and, for a librarian like me who uses her eyes to read and study, that is a long time. I had a lot of astigmatism and then got glasses for it from Dr. Landow, so that enabled me to read as much as I needed to. It was difficult but it all worked out. I did not miss a lot of work and was never incapacitated. If I had my right eye working by then, it would have been even less of a problem.

The Second Surgery in May

Going back for the second surgery, I was even less nervous than I had been the first time. As before, Dr. Price implanted the lens and was able to partially correct the astigmatism. The surgery itself went better from my perspective because I was able to keep my left eye still more than I had the first time.

The whole recovery process took about two months, the same as it had for the first surgery. Once they were convinced that the wound and stitches had healed, I had an office appointment where they removed the stitches. Clipping them relaxed my eye. I think people need to understand that it's not until this point that you approach the final version of what your eyesight is really going to be. It might be two months post-surgery before you experience your best results. It's not like LASIK where you go in and soon thereafter, simply wake up able to see everything.

With both of my eyes, stitches came to the surface and irritated my eyes. The first time, Dr. Kelley clipped all but one of the stitches. The second time it happened on a weekend, of course, and I called Dr. Ali who was on call. He offered to come into the office and clip them on Sunday, but I chose to wait until Monday when Dr. Kelley took care of it quickly. About two weeks ago, the third stitch surfaced and I knew what it was right away. Once again, Dr. Kelley pulled out the stitch and I haven't had any problems since.

The one thing I have noticed is that I can see the top of the lens at night when lights hit my eyes at a certain angle. With eyes like mine, I've had to adjust to coping with many things and so this is a pretty minor issue.

How Life Has Changed

There are simple and profound ways that life has changed for me like just waking up in the morning and being able to see the clock! If I am dressing up, because I don't have to wear glasses all the time, I can go without them. It removes a barrier between the world and me because when I wear glasses people can't see my eyes and my vision hasn't been corrected quite enough for me to ever see facial expressions.

Right now I am a candidate for ordination in the Presbyterian Church and before surgery, when I preached, I couldn't see any further back than the first three rows. In order to be truly effective, I needed to be able to see further than that, and now I can. I can also see my sermon notes better using my glasses. That makes me a more effective and persuasive speaker.

Regarding my personal life, I am a water person: I love the water. Once on vacation in South Florida in the ocean, I got out far enough that I couldn't see which way the shore was. That will not happen to me again now. I can go out swimming and feel confident that I will be able to fully see the environment.

I am so excited for my son, too. He put his first glasses on when he was thirteen months old and he's just never had much time without them. He can have the same surgery I did when he is around 22 years old and I know it will change his life for the better.

I think it's interesting that there is a psychological adjustment to go through when your vision has dramatically improved. I sometimes act as if I can see more than I really can. I have tried hard to make myself understand that when I think I see someone, I actually am seeing who I think it is. In the past, it's been embarrassing when I have mistaken someone. Now I feel sure that will happen less often.

Another thing I find interesting is that in our culture, looks are such a big deal. When I no longer wore "Coke bottle" glasses, I was treated differently. A barrier had been removed and people could more easily see my eyes and my facial expression. We seldom think about how much this affects our interactions with other people. We just tend to take it for granted.

Advice to the Reader

My personal strength and courage come from God and from Nature. I look at the world through my faith so my comments should be read in that context. The miracle in my story is the way that everything came together - circumstances, people and resources. It is truly miraculous that I can wake up in the morning now and see. I can look across a field and see the trees on the other side as individual tree shapes. If we transfer this same process and apply it to people, it helps me relate to others in a way that I simply couldn't before. Having a full set of senses through which to perceive the world has made a very big difference in my life.

To anyone considering surgery on his or her eyes, I would say consider it carefully and trust your instinct as long as that instinct is not fear. It's often difficult to discern: is fear the source of my reluctance? Or does my reluctance come from other sources? If all that is holding you back is fear, then go for it.

There is always a risk in anything you do, and I certainly felt I took an educated risk going into surgery. I acknowledge that it does take a certain amount of courage to go through it. But with God's help and the support of my loving friends and family, I gathered strength enough to do it. I am thankful for their support and that kind of social support network is important to all of us. It is not a reason not to have the surgery, but I would urge patients to gather that support. Don't go forward without talking about it and informing others in your support system of everything you know. Don't try to be a hero; some people go through things stoically and don't discuss it with their employer, for example. If your employer knows the facts and holds realistic expectations, they are able to offer you help and it will always work out better for everyone involved.

I am appreciative that Dr. Price takes things very slowly. It was so helpful that we did only one eye at a time; that gave me time to adjust. I am very grateful to God for living in a time when I could experience this correction before I died. I am indebted to Dr. Landow for being proactive and grateful to Dr. Kelley, Dr. Price and the whole staff for their kindness, their expertise and their willingness to work with me and answer my questions.

I want to close with one additional thought: the mission at the Foundation is quite a wonderful one. I am excited about seeing this book when it is done and I look forward to celebrating its birth with Dr. Price and all of you. Thank you for including me. I hope my story helps others.

Fuchs' Dystrophy

"Tickled Pink"

Claire Brenner is a gentle, passionate woman with a sense of humor that permeates her soft manner of speaking and makes for a delightful conversation. Her spirituality and creativity are linked to a belief that we are all being guided by a Higher Purpose to serve one another and the world with our gifts. The threatened loss of her sight has only deepened that belief with gratitude for having been led to the right people at the right time.

When I was a young child I was diagnosed with far-sightedness and fitted with glasses. I wore them for as long as I can remember so I never gave much thought to them. I understand now that this is a hereditary condition and can be taken care of with a very simple, in-the-office procedure.

It was 15 years ago that I noticed when I was driving my car and I was tired that I would sometimes see double. I'd have to pull over and, eventually, I decided to wear a patch on one eye so that I could manage. It was pretty dangerous and not much of a solution.

Over time, I developed a cataract in my left eye and about three years ago I had it removed. The doctor told me it was the "easiest" cataract removal he had ever done. Unfortunately, my eye began to swell and my vision began to deteriorate. I would call his office to report it and was constantly reassured that the swelling would go down; that is, when I could get them to return my calls. The swelling never went down and everything was a blur in that eye. The doctor just casually said to me one day, "Don't worry; we'll do a corneal transplant." By then I did not have any faith left in this doctor or the surgeon he recommended for my transplant.

Doing My Homework

I called my nephew who has had severe eye problems since childhood and has undergone numerous operations on his eyes. He supposedly has the "best doctor in the country" and so I asked him to ask his doctor to make a referral for me. His physician suggested a female doctor named Sandy Feldman, M.D. in San Diego. I began going to her, but the swelling still didn't go down and then one day she told me she had worked on an experimental study years before where they performed a different kind of corneal transplant called DSEK (Descemet's Stripping with Endothelial Keratoplasty). She said she would do some looking around and find out who was offering it now and where they were located. Dr. Feldman is a specialist in corneal transplants and I greatly valued her input and her guidance.

She called me back two weeks later with the name of Dr. Francis Price in Indianapolis, IN. and the name of another surgeon in a different city who were both doing the surgery. She advised me that if it were her own eye, she would choose Dr. Price because of his greater length of experience with the procedure and his high success rate. I felt like singing, "It's a miracle, it's a miracle!" I made the decision right then to go ahead with it because I had such faith in her, and the description of the procedure sounded perfect for me.

The biggest advantage was the quicker recovery. At age 77, I did not feel I wanted a surgery where I would have to wait a year for stitches to come out, knowing that even when they did, I might still have blurry vision. The idea of having a procedure with a much faster recovery, and no corneal stitches to deal with, meant that I could regain my lifestyle quickly. I didn't want to wait around; I lead an active life. I need my vision to sew and I love to read.

My sister, Sybil, goes to a doctor in New York who is supposedly a very fine "eye man" and he had never even heard of DSEK. Sybil was worried and told me that I should carefully check my facts. But I was committed to go forward without his okay because it sounded so right for me and I had confidence in my own doctor, as well as in Dr. Price.

When I called Sybil to confirm my plans, I told her that my children and I were pooling our money to pay for the surgery. I asked if she would consider contributing, and she declined saying, "No, I want to pay for it all." It was a huge lesson for me in receiving and we are closer now than ever before. She is such a loving, caring person and I am grateful for her compassionate heart and giving spirit.

The Indianapolis Experience

Dr. Price and his staff were generous and sweet with their time, and they made a lot of arrangements that were not necessarily convenient for them. They went out of their way and were extremely helpful to me. (I messed up on the time and we arrived a few days sooner than we should have.) As it turned out, Dr. Price was giving a lecture outside Indiana the weekend right after my surgery and he flew back early on Sunday just to check on me. That gives you an idea of what kind of doctor he is.

Dr. Price is so sweet and dear, very kind and open with his time, not like some doctors who rush you in and out of the office. He is patient no matter how busy he is and that's pretty unusual in my experience. My first impression of him and his team were that they were warm and welcoming. No one kept me waiting, although honestly they could have kept me there all afternoon and I would not have cared. I went there with the attitude that I was very lucky to have found him and everything would work out fine. And it did! I really think the way I found him is a genuine miracle and I think his work is miraculous.

I can now see beautifully! When I left the care of Dr. Price, the double vision persisted as well as a cataract on my right eye. I am going to have prisms ground and put into two pair of eyeglasses so that I won't see double. One pair will be for the farsighted eye and one pair for reading. Then I will be able to drive my car again. It's been over a year since I've been able to drive and I am more than ready to start. It is a joy to have my life back!

I referred another woman to Dr. Price because I am so pleased with my experience. I have not heard from her yet so I don't know if she has decided to have the surgery or how it has turned out. I called my nephew and reported how clearly I could see out of this eye immediately after surgery. I do not wear corrective glasses anymore; I wear a pair with clear lenses only to protect the eye that had surgery. I do not use glasses to read, but I have a pair of inexpensive magnifying glasses from the drug store that I use. My family and I continue to tell everyone we know about my surgery, and the wonderful outcome I had, in order to help spread the word and help others. More doctors need to learn about this procedure and the benefits to their patients.

Each time I have an eye exam for glasses, I can see better and better. I get to read one line lower each time, so my glasses are getting less and less powerful. And isn't that the direction we all want to go?

Life Lessons

I have gained a keener appreciation of my restored sight and, especially, of color. I design and sew a patented system of baby bedding. Part of my success has been due to my use of color, so having my sight again is essential to doing this creative work. Being without the best use of my eyes, there was a point where I thought I could lose them. It was very frightening to me. I did not have enough healing cells behind the cornea and I was in total fear, frankly. I just thank God for whoever donated their cornea to me, and truthfully, I pray for that person, whoever it was, for giving me the gift of sight.

Having time with my daughter, Mara, who accompanied me to Indianapolis for the surgery was a gift that I am grateful for, too. Our time together was wonderful. We had a few days before the surgery and spent hours talking, sharing and shopping. It was very good for our relationship and I consider it a bonus from the trip that will be a lasting memory for us both.

I am not religious, but I am spiritual. I believe in Spirit, a life energy force that is ongoing and all around us. That same electrical energy exists between people and is contained within our speech and in our thoughts. Therefore, I watch what I say and what I think about because I know there is great power in both. I have to admit that I don't always do it as much as I should.

I derive a great deal of strength and courage from my children and grandchildren. They are good human beings! I am proud to know them. My son, Jonathan and my daughter, Mara, are ethical, moral people. My two grandchildren, Alexander and Kylie, are also incredible beings. They will make a difference in the world someday; I am sure of it.

Advice to Readers

It's a difficult thing to give advice. If you are having vision trouble of any kind, can you accept advice from anyone? I am not sure. If we are in fear, we don't hear anything but our fear. And if we are not in fear, we will listen to our Higher Power and work it through the way it should be.

I do want to say thank God for men like Dr. Price; he is an incredible man with such a loving, sweet energy about him. It was a treat to meet him and be with him and with all the people who work with him in his practice. They were so kind to me. I cannot understand why every doctor is not there studying with him, learning this new procedure. He's such a natural teacher and a total delight. My time there was very special.

I also want to mention Dr. Ali who skillfully assisted Dr. Price; I just love him! He's fabulous looking, too! You want your eyes just so you can gaze upon him, and by the way, Dr. Price is no slouch, either! Seriously, I want to say thanks for the opportunity to share my story in the hopes that it might help someone else along their Path. If it helps in any way, I will be tickled pink! This book's a wonderful idea.

Fuchs' Dystrophy

"My Miracle Worker"

Pat Cowan was wearing orange-feathered Halloween earrings and a brightly patterned Halloween sweater when we met for her interview in October. A spirited woman, she clearly likes to have fun, and to enjoy life to the fullest. For many years a legal secretary, Pat has transferred her passion for details into her work as a volunteer helping senior citizens make their way through a maze of healthcare and Medicare questions. Warm and witty, she has a perfect mate in her equally warm and witty husband, Lou, to whom she has been married for 50 years.

I was six years old when I got my first pair of glasses and they were thick ones. I don't remember much about grade school except that I did not want to be assigned a place in the "sight-saving" class. That seemed too drastic and I didn't want to go *there*! So I told my mother that I just wasn't going to go to school at all if that happened, and in the end, I got my way and entered a regular class instead.

Looking back, I can recall my eyes tiring easily and having many reading problems in school. I had a lot of difficulties with depth perception, too; I could hardly see my hands in front of my face. I also had continuing trouble seeing a ring of "circles" around lights, like red and green traffic lights, the sun, and the moon. I just thought everyone saw these objects the way I did. It also seemed that every time I got a new prescription for glasses, I would have to watch where I was going very carefully so I wouldn't stumble and fall.

My mother developed macular degeneration as she aged, and because of that I thought I should see an ophthalmologist for eye exams, instead of an optometrist. The doctor I chose assured me that I did not have the same condition as my mom; but he told me that I had extremely bad astigmatism and that cataracts were starting to form. From 1989 to 2002, my story is typical of what happens to many people with Fuchs' Dystrophy. I went to a different ophthalmologist who did a test for dry eyes, but never mentioned Fuchs' to me. He advised the use of Preservation drops during the daytime and Preservation night ointment that helped. He never mentioned Muro.

I had several bouts with blisters, but never understood what caused them. My doctor never addressed the condition with me, and he just kept insisting that I use the eye drops and the ointment. Whenever I called his office, it seemed as if I always got the same answer: there were no appointments open and I would have to wait until the next day. Then the next day would come and my eye would feel a bit better and, since it was always difficult to get time off work, I would decide not to keep the appointment.

Learning about My Condition

My eyes usually felt like I had sand in them and they often itched. I later found out that the itching was caused by allergies, something else that was never diagnosed or discussed with me. Finally, in sheer frustration with what felt like arrogance in my latest doctor, combined with the lack of help I was getting, I decided to change doctors again. I found an optometrist I liked who was recommended by several friends; once again during the exam I was told that I did not have macular degeneration, but I did have cataracts and a lot of astigmatism.

When I had the next attack of blisters, I stopped in my optometrist's office and he told me to wait because he wanted to examine my eyes. He gave me some numbing drops and an antibiotic. He told me that if I had any more trouble with my eyes, he was going to refer me to an ophthalmologist he would recommend. Blisters, by the way, are miserable. It feels like you have a paper cut in your eye and you just can't get comfortable, no matter how often you blink or what you do.

I was growing tired of living with cataracts and I wanted to do something about them in order to enjoy life more. I decided to see the ophthalmologist who had been recommended; during the exam I was diagnosed with "Fuchs' Dystrophy." It was the first time I had ever heard the term. The doctor told me that he would not operate on my cataracts because he was afraid it would cause the Fuchs' to accelerate. He advised me to use Muro ointment and that helped. He also told me that he did not think I was quite ready yet for a transplant. It was November of 2004.

I went home and got immediately on the Internet to find out all I could about Fuchs'. I read everything I could find on the topic, and I also joined Fuchs Friends, an online chat group and resource site (www.fuchsfriends.com) for people with the condition.

A Disappointment Leads To Hope

I was sure the time had come for me to visit a corneal specialist so, with great hopes, I had my first appointment in January 2005. I explained about the glare, the circles around the lights, the feeling of sand in my eyes, not being able to drive at night, not being able to focus in the morning and needing increasingly stronger magnifying glasses to read. The doctor advised against me having a corneal transplant because he thought I was not "ready" for it.

I was disappointed, but I had done my homework and so I asked him about DLEK. He said "no" to that, too, because he felt it was "too new a procedure." He mentioned that a physician friend of his was working on a three-year study at the Mayo Clinic and when it was completed, he thought he would begin performing DLEK on patients. He had also just opened a new laser clinic and it seemed to me that he was more interested in that than in helping me. Neither Lou nor I were positively impressed with him.

Looking back, this disappointment was actually a good thing because it helped me become really clear about my feelings: I knew I did not want to wait three more years before doing something to improve my vision. I was ready for a change! The people in Fuchs Friends had already told me that Dr. Price was the doctor I should be seeing. I decided to call him for a consultation and it has been one of the best decisions I have ever made. My appointment was in March 2005.

First Impressions

My first impression of Dr. Price and his team was "They are fantastic!" Everybody was just so friendly and made me and Lou feel really comfortable. They were very understanding and I just loved all of them. I knew I was in the right place and I felt great confidence in Dr. Price. I had never been given tests for glare or corneal thickness, but they were part of the work-up. His staff also did several other tests that were new to me. The whole atmosphere in the clinic was so supportive, up-to-date and professional. I learned a lot as I went through the process; it opened new doors of information for me and increased my sense of positive anticipation and eagerness to have the surgery. Finally, after all the doctors I had seen, I had found the right one!

On April 27, I had the first surgery on my right eye to remove the cataracts and have a cornea replacement. The surgery was a breeze and I had no pain whatsoever. Dr. Price always makes me feel calm because he is so matter of fact and calm himself. Dr. Ali, his assistant that day, was great, too, and my husband even took pictures of both of them. Lou later told me that it was like a coffee klatch in the waiting room while I was having surgery. Other family members were waiting for their loved ones, and everyone talked with one another and shared their feelings and their stories. We were among kindred spirits.

The Surgery

Let me briefly explain what the surgery was like and what happened. Many people are afraid of eye surgery, but it is actually a comfortable procedure and nothing to be afraid of. I was given several drops in my eye and then told to wait for awhile before taking me back to the operating suite. In the prep room, I got into a surgical gown and cap and got an IV of a relaxing medication. I went into "la la" land. Lou was with me right up until they administered the anesthetic. I had an injection to freeze the eye and soon after, I got pretty sleepy. I had a softening patch put over the eye. They woke me up as they took me into the surgery room, and I was semi-awake from there on. I could hear Dr. Price's voice and I was aware of what was going on around me. I did not feel a thing; no pain or discomfort at all. At the end of the surgery, Dr. Price put a contact lens in my eye and then I was wheeled into the recovery room.

We stayed overnight at a local hotel nearby and I had to lie on my back all night. I had an early appointment the next day; Dr. Price examined my eye to make sure the air bubble pressing against the cornea was still in place. We came back the second day for another exam and I was amazed at how well I could see! Three big E's on the visual acuity chart and the whole first line! He released me to go home and wanted me to have follow-up with my optometrist.

I rested quite a bit that first week after surgery, and I also had my first check-up with my doctor. He monitored my eye drops and started me on PredForte and then removed the contact lens two weeks after surgery. After four months, my vision was 20/25, the best I have ever seen in that eye since I can't remember when.

More on the Horizon

I am still not done; I have another surgery scheduled for my left eye for cornea transplant and cataract removal. I can hardly wait to see the results. I have told everyone I know that I think Dr. Price is a miracle worker. I would recommend his practice, Price Vision Group, to anyone and everyone that needs help. Everyone on his staff is so caring and thorough in their examinations. You are in good hands with them.

I am at an age to be considered a senior citizen now and I want to travel with my husband, Lou. By the way, I have decided to say that I am only 29 years old. After all, age is only a number by which to judge my experience! I celebrate each year as another "anniversary" of turning 29! (Jack Benny celebrated being 39, but I think women ought to be allowed to be a bit younger.)

When Lou and I go on trips now, I can see all the colors of the trees and the sky. I can see the faces of my grandkids clearly. I can thread a needle again and have taken up my sewing after not being able to do it for ten years. I can focus my eyes and read the daily newspaper again; it has been so hard to see for such a long time that it's just great to be alive!

The most important lesson I have learned from regaining my sight is an appreciation for the gift of vision. It has enabled me to volunteer again for something I love: being able to help senior citizens. I volunteer for seniors in Illinois helping them with their medical bills and insurance questions. Some of these people are surviving on such a small amount of money that it makes you wonder how they can live. I am so glad I can offer help that makes a practical difference in their lives. Without my sight, I would not be able to do this work.

Advice to Readers

My advice is if you have eye troubles, go for help now! The longer you wait, the worse it will get. Do it now! It will feel like opening a door into a new world. Any discomfort you have will soon be gone and there's no sense in waiting. If you get ten years of improved vision from it, isn't that worth it?

I would also say "reach out" to other people for support. For those readers who have Fuchs' Dystrophy, there's a great group called "Fuchs' Friends." This is one of the nicest group of people you could ever know. For example, one woman I met there had breast cancer last year and she said later that she could not have gotten through it if it hadn't been for the support of the people in Fuchs' Friends. We are a great collection of people and I would like to directly say "thank you" to everyone in the organization. Without your website and your knowledge, love and loyal support, I would never have found Dr. Price, my miracle worker.

I'll close by saying that my inspiration in life comes from God, Lou, my great husband of 50 years, my two dear daughters and five beautiful grandchildren, my caring family and friends and my deep love for the beauty of nature. My philosophy of life is this: if something can be done, I want to do it. I know that Dr. Price is the same way and that's why he keeps finding new solutions and is able to help so many people.

Fuchs' Dystrophy

"Beautiful!"

Donald Wright is a man who speaks in measured phrases; he is thoughtful and naturally tells a story thoroughly with details and dates. His easy laughter balances the logic with which he describes the events that led up to his corneal transplant and the impact it's made on his life.

Mine is a story of a gradual decline in my vision over a period of years. The first time I really noticed that I had a problem was when I was sitting at my desk one day in my early 40's. I had been trying to read an article, and I had been reading and re-reading and I couldn't seem to get anywhere when I suddenly realized that I couldn't *see* it. I went to Dr. Irving Gurwood, my ophthalmologist, to have an eye exam and that's when I got my first reading glasses. Prior to this episode, I had not had any vision problems whatsoever so I regarded it as a normal problem of middle age.

My vision continued to gradually decline until fifteen years ago when I noticed that, even with a new pair of corrected glasses, I still had trouble seeing some things like the golf ball when I was out playing golf with friends. I began telling Dr. Gurwood that I couldn't understand why he was unable to correct my vision more. Even with new glasses, my vision was never corrected totally and it puzzled and frustrated me. As I approached retirement, I realized something else was going on. It got to the point that when I played golf I had to have someone stand behind me because I had no idea where the ball was going. My eyes couldn't follow the ball at all.

Finally, Dr. Gurwood diagnosed me with Fuchs' Dystrophy and began treating it with an eye ointment. He made me aware of what I should expect including the fact that eventually I would need surgery. It was a relief to have a diagnosis, but the ointment didn't enhance my vision. In fact, no matter what we did, we couldn't seem to correct the situation. We decided to just watch it and do what we could in the meantime.

Search for the Best

It wasn't long after my diagnosis that Dr. Gurwood heard of this new corneal transplant procedure which I later learned was being done by Dr. Price. I knew something had to be done because my vision was increasingly getting worse. I read a few articles about the procedure and it was obviously superior to other treatments. The recovery time was better, and the time it took to achieve improved vision was shorter than a standard transplant. My doctor was very high on the procedure and enthusiastic about me having the surgery when I felt ready.

It was two years ago, at the age of seventy, when I finally reached the point where I was ready for surgery, and I began contacting surgeons in my area who were familiar with the new procedure.

As my conducted my research, I found a few local doctors who were using the new procedure. But when I looked more closely, I found they had done very few of these surgeries with only a low rate of success. I started to get nervous about it. Even though I had been referred to an excellent eye center and had found a very good surgeon, I wasn't satisfied it was the best I could do. The surgeon that I had chosen was excellent and had undergone some training with Dr. Price. When I discussed my concerns with him, however, he assured me that if I had any misgivings at all, I should contact Dr. Price for a consultation. I took his sage advice and learned that Dr. Price had done hundreds of these new procedures and had a success rate up in the nineties. I felt very confident that I had found the best, and I made arrangements to have the surgery in Indianapolis with him in August 2004.

Looking back, I was, and still am, grateful that both of my local doctors were instrumental in helping me find the best person and place to have it done. The center where I was referred was renowned for excellence but they just were not up to speed on this procedure yet. I am grateful for the wise guidance and cooperation I got and have nothing but praise for them both. They put my needs and my care first.

Indianapolis Experience

My first impression was very favorable of Dr. Price and his staff. It is one of the best-organized medical clinics I've ever visited, if not the best. Everyone was very friendly, helpful and cooperative. They seemed to know their jobs and did them very well. I was impressed with the whole organization, especially Dr. Price. He was relaxed, competent, and seemed focused and interested in me. My wife, Ann, was also very impressed with the whole organization from the minute we walked in until we left. They made us both feel welcome; they were efficient and we could tell we were in the best place for us to be. We knew they were going to help us.

I went in on a Monday and I had a thorough eye exam. When I was asked to read the wall chart with my left eye, all I could see was the light on the wall, and nothing else. Two days later I had surgery and came out with a patch on my eye. It was a quick and painless procedure.

I followed the post-operative instructions to lie flat for 24 hours and then come back to see Dr. Price the next day. When they removed the eye patch, I was amazed because my vision was immediately improved. I could read several lines down on the chart without any correction. It was miraculous. When Dr. Price examined my eye, he looked up at me and said,

"Beautiful!" Ever since that moment, this became my favorite word in the English language. He called in his associates and they had superlative things to say as well. It made me feel wonderful.

Ann could not fully appreciate what I was going through because her own vision is good, but she had watched me struggling for so long and the results were just amazing. We knew my vision would improve with surgery, but we did not know it was going to be an immediate improvement.

Since then, I have had several examinations in different clinics and all the doctors have said things like "terrific" and "amazing." They are all impressed with the work and with the condition of my eye. It has felt so good to receive this affirmation of my restored sight.

How Life Has Changed

I went back to normal life right away. I just had a few minor restrictions but nothing major. I could not bend over, for example, to tie my shoelaces nor was I allowed to lift anything heavy. I had to rest a bit more than usual. The whole recuperation period was several weeks in length while I observed these minor restrictions. It was a fast improvement and an easy recovery.

In the important ways, though, my life changed a great deal after the surgery. For example, one of my hobbies is playing a trombone in a brass group at my church. I had been forced to memorize my music because I couldn't see it well. Now I can see the music again and it makes playing a whole lot easier! Also, I can now follow a golf ball better; the vision in my left eye is so good it compensates for the weakness in my right eye. And reading is now possible again. I had been using a large print Bible because I couldn't see regular size print.

In addition, driving my car has returned; I can even drive at night again. When I get the other eye done, it will be even better. It's funny but that eye had been my "best" eye before the surgery. Now I know it has to be done because the vision is quite blurred. I just have to decide when I want to have it done and make those plans. I think it will be within the next two years.

There's another change that I have made since having the surgery. I think we all have a tendency to take things for granted but I appreciate my blessings now more than ever. I certainly appreciate the fact that some people are devoting their lives to helping others like Dr. Price is doing. He is a humble man, down to earth, but he has this tremendous gift. I truly appreciate the research he's doing. I donate to his Foundation because he is so impressive to me and he is using his gift to benefit mankind.

Advice to Readers

If you are considering eye surgery, do it! You could look the world over and you wouldn't find anyone more qualified than Dr. Price. But if you don't live in the United States, or don't want to travel to Indianapolis, then find a top notch, quality doctor in your area with lots of experience and a good success rate. The procedure is good, so all you have to do is find the right doctor. I would also suggest finding other people who have gone through the same experience as you have because it will strengthen you to talk with them, and will help reduce any fear you may have.

One other thing I want to say is that, unfortunately, sometimes as you get older you are reminded of your age and rather than hearing what can be done to help you, you are discouraged from seeking help. Reject this approach. Find a doctor who wants to help you. You're never too old for good sight.

I have drawn strength and courage from my good wife, Ann, from my family and from close friends. It is my belief and faith in God that continually strengthens and inspires me. There is no better source of courage and wisdom than that.

Fuchs' Dystrophy

"Gutsy Up!"

I first "met" Doris Hinderliter through a letter she wrote to Dr. Price after her corneal transplant surgery in the summer of 2005. (Her letter is included at the end of this chapter.) Her straightforward, no nonsense approach was heartening and her story was earlier descried in Visionary, the Foundation's quarterly newsletter. An artist, Doris' perspective on life reflects her love of beauty, balance and the Original Creator.

Up until 18 months ago, as far as I knew, I did not have an eye problem. I had worn eyeglasses for reading but it was not imperative so sometimes I didn't even bother wearing them. I didn't have a vision problem but I did have terrible dry eyes now and then, and I noticed I had begun to have trouble with night driving in the past few years. But I had never heard the words "Fuch's Dystrophy" until I developed terrible blisters on my eyes. It happened suddenly, out of the blue, and the pain was excruciating and horrible. Two weeks later, I had an emergency standard corneal transplant and I am still having problems with it compared with the more recent cornea-sparing surgery Dr. Price performed on my other eye in June of this year.

I regularly visit the Fuchs' Friends website (www. fuchsdystrophy.com) and I have read comments by so many people struggling with the decision to have a transplant and I just can't relate to it. When I was in agony, I wanted help of any kind; having a transplant was a welcome choice even though it was scary. I was in such pain I didn't care what was done. I wanted relief.

I learned about Dr. Price through Fuchs' Friends; members talk among themselves and offer the names of surgeons who are the most skilled. I considered going to a doctor in Portland, but Dr. Price is in the Midwest, and I am from the Midwest, so that sounded good to me. I also used their website resources to compare various surgical methods. I liked the description of the advanced corneal transplant, the new posterior graft procedure, so that was another easy decision. Finally, the folks on the website talked about how wonderful a doctor he is. I sensed Dr.Price was going to be the right doctor for me. I called and got an appointment, had my records sent and then traveled to Indianapolis with my daughter, Jane.

My first impressions of Dr. Price and the clinic staff was that they were very warm, very caring, and that it was a nice environment and a great organization. I had not had the same impressions elsewhere; I had been yanked around a bit. As I spent time with Dr. Price and his team, I thought to myself, "I must have come to the right place if they can be this considerate and this humane." Jane was equally impressed with the treatment; she had been to other places with me and she could tell the difference, too. (Jane is likely to be a future Fuchs' dystrophy patient herself some day.)

My Surgery

I had a great deal of faith in Dr. Price as I went into surgery. I had no worry about it at all. My surgery went smoothly. Dr. Price and his staff were very considerate and I loved having it done in the same building. That was an advantage. The clinic setting was much less frightening than going into some huge edifice of a public hospital. To be able to just go downstairs into the operating suite in the same building was great. In my case, I didn't want to be exposed to all the germs in a hospital and did not want the sheer inconvenience of it.

Each of Dr. Price's team contributed to making me feel at ease and safe. They answered my questions and there were many friendly faces around me as I was prepared for surgery and during the procedure. I did not feel as if I were among strangers who were going to do things to me that would hurt. From the receptionist to the woman who counted the cells, all were friendly and kind. I have had two transplants so I can compare both experiences and this one was definitely the better of the two.

All I remember about the surgery is seeing colors; I must have been under anesthesia but I saw lovely, soothing images of colors. It was very pleasant. The surgery itself was a bloodless surgery; people should not be afraid of it. It's quite a tidy, clean and brief process, not like having major surgery with big bandages such as a hysterectomy, for example. It is not frightening and it is fast. The only recommendation I have to make it even better would be to play some soft classical music in the clinic during the preparation phase.

Post-surgery, I never had a "real" recuperation; compared to my other eye surgery, it was a miracle because I noticed an *immediate* improvement. With my other surgery, I had constant pain. By comparison, during the week I spent in Indy and after I returned home, I did not feel a bit of pain. I had to lie still on my back for 24 hours afterwards but that was a small restriction to endure. I was quite willing to do anything and determined to follow all the instructions.

To be able to see so well after only one week is a miracle. I believe my sight is a gift of God given to me through Dr. Price. Having my vision restored has given me hope, and so much of my lifestyle has been given back to me. I am an artist and my artwork is vital to me. I had to give it up as my sight failed but now I am back once more sculpting, making jewelry and enameling on copper – a lot of my work involves fine and intricate things. I have been making silver jewelry for many years, and you can see an example that I am wearing in the photograph. That necklace happens to be made of many

47

sawn pieces of silver bent to link together by hooking one piece upon another without use of chain links or solder as is usually done. I also enjoy setting stones into handmade bezels, forming shapes by repousse (hammering heated metal) into original designs and interesting forms of sculpture. I like to combine this with glass enameled copper which I also craft.

I spent many long years perfecting my skills. I am so grateful that I do not have to give it all up. The corneal transplant has enabled me once more to get back to doing the creative work I enjoy. I am also a bookworm and now I can read with glasses, even if it's not for long periods of time. I feel so fortunate.

Advice to Readers

Keep the faith. Things can get better. Keep an open mind; study and learn as much as you can and continue to be informed so you can make good decisions. Knowledge is power! I wish there had been more time before I had to make the decision to have my first eye done; I might have been able to find Dr. Price and have the new cornea-sparing procedure instead.

Do your homework and look for a doctor who is intelligent, inquiring, and someone who hasn't "retired" while still on the job. Look for enthusiasm, someone who continues to find new and better ways to do his work and who has the patient's best interests at heart. It is equally important to have someone with a good deal of experience. I think Dr. Price is this kind of doctor. I also think this book is a great way for the Foundation to get the word out and help doctors and patients understand what it's like to live with vision challenges and how new procedures can bring significant improvements to the quality of life.

One other thing: when you have only one eye corrected and not the other, you lose depth perception. It's dangerous, especially for people who are older, because you can easily fall. For people contemplating vision surgery, safety from falling should be an important consideration. I also think ophthalmologists lack awareness of how important this factor is and they should be helped to better understand that falling is a serious problem for the elderly.

My own strength comes from my faith in God. Like all of us, I have had my share of life's trials and tribulations. I would have to say that my greatest inspiration is my mother's example of how she lived and looked at life. She raised three kids during the Depression after my Dad died. He left no insurance because it had lapsed for lack of money, and here she was alone with this huge responsibility. I was not yet six years old; my sister was three and my brother was twelve. My Mom had no skills and had never worked. It was very rough but never once were we on welfare. She was a beacon of courage; she worked and taught us to always do our best, to be brave and to keep going. She taught us to believe that things will work out and you will be led to the very best places and people if you are truly serious about finding them.

I was able to put myself through college; my siblings also went to college and we all graduated. We had this family expression to "gutsy up" and it meant to get yourself together and just do it. Courage was being afraid and doing it anyway. Telling yourself, I can do this, I must do this, I will do this! Whining was not permitted.

I had cancer five years ago and it's in remission now. Just as I did with regard to my vision, I read all I could find; I looked closely at all the doctors, and kept my head to make an informed decision. I was scared, but knowledge always makes us stronger. I hope this book will make many people stronger and I wish you could send a copy to every ophthalmologist's office.

Postscript: Here is Doris' letter reprinted as it was received:

Dear Dr. Price,

Just a note to say how thrilled I am to be painlessly looking through the very clear "window on the world" you built for me on June 8, 2005! The DSEK (new cornea-sparing transplant) has far exceeded my hopes - it has been completely painless since the end of week one. This is in such contrast to the year long, often severe, discomfort I experienced in the traditional transplant done 3/04 in the other eye. Vision in the DSEK eye is now much better than in the traditional transplant eye and has greatly improved my depth perception. I have not stumbled or fallen since getting it - a real "plus" in the safety department and a fact that is seldom mentioned anywhere.

I know Dr. Rouweyha said he would call you to report the 10% progress made in the unhealed area of my eye, etc but I wanted to write this to express my sincere appreciation for your work and for the kindness and consideration shown to me (as well as to my daughter Jane, who accompanied me) by you and your entire staff. Thank you again.

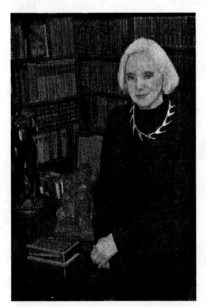

Sincerely,
Doris Hinderliter

Credits:

Photography by Michelle Evans and Edie Chiarappa
Hair, makeup, and styling by Edie Chiarappa

Aniridia

"It's Not New York!"

The Cruz family interview took place by phone on a Saturday morning. Ray Cruz, a New York City detective of 20 years, and his wife, Linda, are warm, enthusiastic and genuine people. The sense of hope they feel was palpable as they described their medical journey with their six year-old son, Michael, who was born without irises. Grateful for the help they received from The Lighthouse program and from Dr. Price and his staff, their courage and faith are representative of loving parents the world over who seek the best for their children. (The story is written from Linda's perspective.)

Michael was born at 38 weeks by C-section; he was a healthy baby, who weighed 7 pounds, 7 ounces. No one told us anything was wrong with him when he was in the hospital. We thought he was perfect just like our first-born son, Eric. We noticed that they put some white gel in his eyes but they told us they did that with all new babies. They checked him out and released us both with no special instructions.

Five weeks after I had him, I took him with me to visit my sister, Liza, in Florida. Almost immediately, she noticed there was something wrong with Michael's eyes; he didn't focus properly, the lights bothered him and his eyes were always moving. She insisted something was wrong and I got scared. I started wondering if his eyes were the problem or if there was something else wrong, like autism. I had read about autistic children who lived in their own world and I was worried that it might be the reason why he was not interacting with me. I just didn't know what to do at first, but I kept praying.

We returned home on a Sunday and the next day had an emergency appointment with our pediatrician, Dr. Malva. She examined Michael and told us straight out, "He does not have irises." I asked her if she thought he could also be autistic and she reassured me that he was not. She then rushed us to see an eye specialist in Great Neck, New York that same day.

Unfortunately, this doctor did not have a good bedside manner; he depressed us by telling us that Michael was blind without irises and would be "handicapped" for the rest of his life. He did not offer us any help in understanding aniridia, the name for the condition Michael has, so in a sense we were blind, too. A short time later we got a letter from the New York State Commission for the Blind; the law requires doctors to report babies that are blind and that's how we learned that Michael had been declared legally blind. It was a dark period for us as a family.

I went through so much depression with Michael; I thought God had let me down. I still get emotional talking about how I felt. We had already been through a frightening experience four years earlier with our first-born, Eric. He was only eight months old when he rolled off our bed onto a parquet floor and developed a blood clot on his brain. He almost passed away on us and it was such a blessing that he survived without any lingering health concerns. He is now a bright, healthy, and happy ten-year old "Big Brother" to Mike.

It was not until we saw a third specialist, Dr. Kaufmann, that we began to learn about aniridia. She was more informative and sympathetic to what we were going through as Michael's parents than the previous doctor was. She told us that it was a rare condition, and taught us what to do and what not to do. Our expectations began to change and we felt more hopeful.

The Lighthouse

Michael was about seven months old when Dr. Malva referred us to The Lighthouse for early intervention services. They sent a team to our home to evaluate his needs. There were four different therapists on the team who saw him: an occupational, a physical, a speech and a visual therapist. They were just the best of the best! They worked with him seven days a week in our home. When they began he couldn't even sit up. On a changing table he couldn't roll over. He did not have any body strength and his muscles were weak. They explained to us why this happens: when babies are blind they cannot tell where their body is in space. They don't have visual cues from their environment to help them balance and so they tend to be inactive and their muscles are under- used.

As the therapy team began making regular home visits, we saw immediate improvements in Michael. We watched them as they played with him and helped him start to catch up with normal development. They were wonderful. Lighthouse International is located on 59th Street and Lexington Avenue in New York City.

As a result of their interventions, he was walking by the age of one and we found that amazing. Even some sighted kids don't walk until they are 14-15 months old! I don't know how they did it even though I sat with them and watched them work. They were excellent and so skillful in getting him to respond.

At the age of three, Mikey started attending their preschool and it was a great place for him. He has continued there and he loves his teachers and the daily routine. We think it's terrific that he does his homework so earnestly and never wants to disappoint them. In fact, sometimes we joke that we wish we had as much influence on him!

Finding Dr. Price

Just as Michael was learning to cope with his challenges, we were reading everything we could get our hands on about aniridia on the Internet. Then, about two years ago, Dr. Kaufmann read an article by Dr. Price and told us about an iris implant surgery he was doing. She told us that Michael would never have 20/20 vision, but he could be helped by artificial iris implants and they would make a real difference in his life. We figured it was better to do something than to do nothing. In fact, by the time we left her office that day, we had decided to contact Dr. Price and go all the way with it.

We were prepared to make it happen even if our insurance plan would not cover the expenses of the procedure. For example, Ray had always wanted a Corvette and four years before he had purchased a showroom condition car that was his pride and joy. He told me that he had decided to sell it so we could use the money to pay off some bills and have it available in case we needed it to get the procedure done. I remember the day that car left our home in a big truck, and, oh his face! I recall how sad he looked. I just couldn't say anything to him because I felt so sorry for him and I was so moved by his actions. The new owner has a small website and every now and then Ray goes and takes a look to see if he has posted any new pictures of the car. He says that he does not feel badly about it and he is planning on purchasing a newer one sometime in the future. As he says, "You do what you have to when it comes to your kids. I have no regrets."

We drove to Indianapolis and met Dr. Price in the spring of 2004. He was candid and told us that Michael would be the youngest child ever to receive an iris implant and he was not sure the FDA would approve it. They had made exceptions for three other children, but all were older than Michael was. He told us there would be a wait for several months, or longer, as his office staff worked on it and began correspondence with our insurance company.

Our first impression of Dr. Price and his staff was great. We loved him! The whole environment was so different from how things were done in New York. The way he and his staff examined Michael and the caring they showed for us was so wonderful. They were very professional. We said to each other, "This is not New York!" We were in shock and asked our selves, "How can they all be this nice?"

We returned home and waited nervously, praying and hoping that it would somehow come together. Months passed and then finally the call came that we'd been waiting for. Dr. Kelley told us that the FDA had made another exception and approved Michael's implant for one of his eyes! We scheduled the first surgery for January 31, 2005. We were both so excited!

The Indianapolis Experience

It took us about 15 hours to drive to Indianapolis and we understood that history was being made with this surgery. We even had a little bit of celebrity because Tony Sterrette, Dr. Price's practice manager, got segments of the forty-five minute procedure filmed by two local television stations. (Tony was wonderful and we can't say enough about him.) They taped Michael going into surgery, interviewed us briefly and then returned the next day to see how he was doing. The video clips were shown on the nightly news and they gave us a copy to take home. We have shown that clip to many friends and family members. Michael's story has touched a lot of hearts.

The surgery went smoothly and Michael's improvement was immediate. That night after surgery, when Ray removed the patch off Mike's eye, he took him out of the hotel room to take a good look at it. (I was too nervous to do it myself, or to even look at the eye.) Michael surprised Ray by telling him he could see a building outside the window across the highway! Later that day, when we were in the car going out to eat, Michael spotted a plane in the sky and pointed it out to us. As we drove, he called my attention to a Hummer going by us and said he could see it clearly. He was so excited by seeing the world without blurriness for the first time in his life, and it touched us.

We have a lot of good memories from our two visits to Indianapolis. For example, one night during our first stay, we went to a Macaroni Grill restaurant and made friends with a waitress there. She was so kind to us that we wrote a letter about her to the company. Michael even got kissed there! We were amazed because you don't get that treatment in New York City. We were recognized and well treated no matter where we went. We were so impressed with everyone in Indiana; they were just great people, so warm and friendly.

Dr. Price applied for approval to do the second implant and it was granted that winter. We came back in February 2005 for the surgery. Going through it a second time was much easier on us. Even the long drive was better because Ray bought a DVD player for the car and the boys actually enjoyed the ride. We felt more secure the second time around and looked forward to being with Dr. Price and his staff again because they were such nice people.

How Life Has Changed

I feel less pressure; we both feel like Michael is going to live a normal life. He likes cars, just like his Dad, and maybe there will be a chance for him to get a driver's license. He really wants to drive and we remember how that first doctor told us to forget about it. He said Mike would never be able to drive a car. But we have hope now. We understand that another aniridia patient, a woman named Trish Zorn, has gotten her license and that is such encouraging news.

The greatest life lesson we have learned is not to be selfish and to treasure what we have in our family. My husband always used to think about work, work, and more work. He was always striving to make more money and planning a second job. He was full of plans and thinking about it every day. After what happened to Michael, he has changed. And I have, too. We both think about the kids first now. We have both matured so much. There are more important things in life than financial worries.

Our son Eric has been impacted, too, and he wrote a composition for school about his experiences with Michael's surgeries. The school liked it so much they made it into a big poster that hung in the school lobby last year for everyone to read. We were so proud of him! He's a great big brother and he really looks out for Michael.

We believe in God and we think that He sent Michael to us for a reason. We were given him to take care of and to do the best for him that we can. It makes us very grateful and appreciative of life.

Advice to Readers & Final Thoughts

If there's a surgery that can help you, don't even think twice. Go for it! It's going to bring you a whole new world and you will see much better. Don't be scared. Be confident in your doctor and have faith.

We draw strength and courage from within our family. Sacrifices have to be made and you do the best you can. We work together, we plan together and we go everywhere together. We are so blessed and we love one another; we are lucky to have these two wonderful, normal boys. In the future more technology will be available so who knows what that might bring?

Ray wrote to Oprah last year to suggest that Dr. Price be featured. It would make a wonderful story to show people the kind of work he is doing to help so many people like us. He has made a huge difference in our lives.

We especially want to congratulate the teachers at PS 21, and especially Ms. Dulitz. She is an inspiration to everyone! She has done wonders for Michael in the Visual Aid program. I have to say she is the best teacher he has ever had! She's tough, but she's great! He has spelling tests on Fridays and he always comes home with 100's all the time. We are in shock with the vocabulary he's learning because he's only in the first grade! She is so caring that when he's sick and doesn't go to school, she calls me up and checks on us. She gave me her home number (which teachers just don't do) and she has encouraged me to call her anytime to talk about Michael's work.

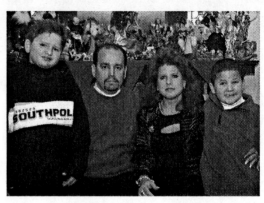

The Cruz Family

Author note:

I briefly spoke with Michael after his parents called him away from the Saturday morning TV shows he was watching. Here's how it went:

EV: Hi, Michael, how are you?

A: *Good.*

EV: I work with Dr. Price and your Mom and Dad have just told me about what happened to you. We're going to put your story in a book. Can you see better since you had the surgery?

A: *Yes, I can. How is Dr. Price?*

EV: He's doing fine, thank you. He went to India and Nepal.

A: *Ok.*

EV: He visited his daughter there and spent Christmas in Nepal.

A: *Wow. That's good. Goodbye!*

Note:

Since 1905, Lighthouse International (www.lighthouse.org) has been the leader worldwide in helping people who are blind or partially sighted overcome the challenges of vision loss. Dedicated to preventing the disabling effects of uncorrectable vision loss from conditions such as macular degeneration, diabetes-related eye disease, cataracts and glaucoma, their work enables people of all ages who are visually impaired to remain independent, active and productive.

The Lighthouse helps people of all ages with vision loss live better by:

- Providing visual rehabilitation services (counseling and training to improve day-to-day functioning)

- Educating eyecare and vision rehabilitation professionals, along with the general public

- Conducting vision, psychosocial, evaluation and accessibility research that provides practical solutions for everyday living

- Promoting the early detection and prevention of vision loss

- Urging policy change through advocacy to ensure equal access to health care, the environment and information

Aniridia

"Gold Medal Advocate"

Trisha ("Trish") Zorn is a woman with a seemingly endless supply of energy. She is the most decorated Paralympian athlete in the history of the games, winning 54 medals, 41 of them gold. She was also a four-time All-American at the University of Nebraska and the first visually impaired athlete to earn a Division 1 scholarship. Winning is in her nature. Trish has overcome barriers that might have been overwhelming because she has been visually impaired from the time she was six months old. Instead, she has chosen to defy the barriers and convert them into opportunities for growth.

My eye condition is called aniridia and I was born with it. The colored part of the eye called the iris was missing in both eyes. I also had cataracts, which typically occur with the condition. It's like having a camera with the lens always open. The light coming in is too strong, plus you are prone to glaucoma because pressure can build up in the eye. Aniridia is a rare condition; when I was first diagnosed at six months of age very little was understood about it because no research had been done.

We now know that aniridia is caused when a dysfunctional gene responsible for eye growth prematurely stops the eye from developing. To get a sense of what it's like, imagine how it feels when you've left a movie theatre after a few hours of sitting in the dark and then stepped into bright sunlight. It makes your eyes tear up and causes you to squint until your eyes adjust to the light. With aniridia, my eyes could not reduce the glare from any source of light and I was unable to see objects further than a few feet away from me. Without irises, I was unable to distinguish colors. Most troubling, my eyes did not have a natural appearance.

When I was nine, my eye doctor tried to fit me with tinted hard contacts in order to eliminate some of the light coming in. They did not fit correctly and actually squeezed my eyes, even though I would wear them for a week and then take them out for a week. They were uncomfortable, and, after a two-month trial we agreed that I would discontinue wearing them.

Going through school was not a very pleasant experience for me. At the time, inclusion of those with disabilities was not a common theory or practice in school systems. I can remember my Mom having to go down to the school district and fight for things like large print books just to give me a level playing field with all the other kids. We always had to ask for special equipment; no one ever just offered it.

From the second grade until I graduated from Mission Vijeo High School in California, I attended Special Education classes. In elementary school it meant that I was pulled out of the regular curriculum for about an hour a day. I was taught practical life skills, like Braille and typing that would benefit me as an adult. But the older I got the less I wanted to be singled out that way due to peer pressure. I didn't want to be made to feel different.

An example that sticks out in my memory happened during a High School English class; I asked my teacher if I could copy her notes and was told "No, that would be cheating." I couldn't see the board, and I wasn't given any other assistance, so it forced me to rely on auditory learning. It was a difficult challenge to overcome, but it taught me to listen carefully and write fast!

A New World Opens

When I was growing up, I also became interested in sports, and participated with enthusiasm in cross-country, track and swimming. Around the age of ten, I got serious about competitive swimming as a member of the Mission Viejo Matadors. From there I went up through the levels to age group swimming, the Junior Nationals, the Nationals, the World Championship trials and, finally, the Olympic trials.

I was sixteen when an article about me appeared in the local newspaper. Two people that were involved with blind and disabled sports called my home and invited me to participate in the National Championship for the Blind being held in Seattle. I did not know much about them and had them confused briefly with the Special Olympics that are for mentally handicapped participants who are not trained athletes. In those games, everyone wins a medal because the primary purpose is socialization. By contrast, Paralympic sports are modeled after the International Olympics. Competitions are held for physically handicapped athletes who have trained hard in certain sports. Their training is often done against able-bodied peers, but the games themselves are competitions held with disabled peers. Only the best three athletes in each sport win the gold, silver and bronze medals.

My parents were protective of me and reluctant to allow me to compete against disabled athletes because I had always competed against those who were sighted. They had sheltered me although they never held me back and they always let me make up my own mind. I was curious about the Championship and so I decided to participate to see what other disabled athletes were like. I had never been around them and I didn't know. My coach allowed me to go up to Seattle and compete and then rejoin my team the next day because we had a meet that same weekend.

It was a transforming experience for me. I realized that it doesn't matter if you have a disability. It doesn't mean anything because it's only a stereotype to think that handicapped people can't excel at sports. When someone tells me that I can't compete because of my disability, they have just lit a fire! No one tells me that I can't do something; I will find a way to do it in order to prove them wrong.

Disabled athletes share a common platform and that is to compete, to challenge themselves and see how far they can push their bodies regardless of their disabilities. They support one another to achieve these goals and they are a tight-knit team. It was very inspiring for me to experience this strength.

I met a lot of people that weekend who shared the same attitude as I have. It just seems so clearly a choice: you can make your disability a positive or a negative thing. I like to describe it this way: my disability has been a *gift* to me. I would not be the same person I am today if I was not born disabled. I might not have been challenged in everyday things; it has made me a stronger person and made me want to succeed more. On every level, I have been challenged by this gift. A disabled person can choose to see their disability as a gift and make something positive out of it, or they can see it as a burden and become filled with self-pity. No one is going to seek you out to help you just because you are disabled. In fact, if you're a negative person, others will avoid you and if you don't get onboard, you will be left behind. That is just the way life is.

That weekend opened a new world to me, and I became intensely involved in Paralympic swimming competitions. In the Olympic Trials for the 1980 Games, I was made the first alternate so I was $1/100^{th}$ away from being chosen for the American team that year. At the time, no "disabled" athlete in any sport had ever made it into the Olympic Games. Since then, a good friend of mine, a distance runner, made the 2000 Games which is a great accomplishment that I celebrate.

When I came into the Games, visually impaired athletes were strong but the competition wasn't deep. It's been nice to see the progression. I've seen it grow and I have been pleased to be part of it. I have been very fortunate to set records; I still hold six world records. In total, I won 55 Paralympic competitive swimming medals from 1980-2004: 41 Gold, 9 Silver and 5 Bronze.

Ever since that time, I have promoted disabled sports quite a lot. I sit on two committees within U.S.A. Swimming, and in the last eight years the level of participation and the desire to implement programs for adapted swimming has really grown. Many people and organizations have been open to discussion and we have all realized that giving opportunities to athletes with disabilities doesn't require a lot. I have been on each side of the discussion table: as an athlete and as an advocate.

About a year ago we started a new program in partnership with the military. We are always looking for new athletes to join our organization and, unfortunately, many of our soldiers in Iraq and other countries have been wounded and disabled. Many were wonderful athletes before they joined the service, and most have never heard of the Paralympic Games. Through our collaboration, these young men and women are hearing about the Games through Walter Reed, Bethesda and other hospitals' Rehabilitation Departments. We have held seminars for them and shown them that they can continue to have sports in their lives. Their adaptations include prosthetics and a lot of training. Many new athletes have joined our ranks, as the result. More information about this program and the organization can be found on the website: www.usparalympics.org

College Experience leads
To a Teaching Career

Because of my athletic background, many different colleges recruited me in my senior year of high school. As I evaluated each one, I considered their academic and athletic programs and the adaptive services they offered disabled students. The University of Nebraska turned out to be a good choice for me, and I am very pleased that I selected them.

Going to college was the first time I had been away from home and Nebraska wasn't too far away (not clear across the country) but still far enough that I felt like I was on my own, which was important to my development. At the University, I also first encountered a department whose mission was to advocate for disabled students on campus. It was called the Office of Adaptive Studies. They helped disabled students in many different ways but primarily they created an inclusive campus experience and ensured that everyone had a fair shot at success, regardless of their disability.

I chose a double major in Elementary and Special Education. I chose Special Ed because of my first-hand experience and the desire to make a difference in that area. On a more personal side, I knew what had worked for me and I knew some things that hadn't work well. I thought if I could make changes based on what I had personally learned, it would make a lasting difference and help many young people.

I chose Elementary Ed because I had been inspired by a great role model, my paternal grandmother, who had been a teacher in the inner city schools of Los Angeles. I can remember her enthusiastically talking about her work and the creative ways she helped students become motivated to learn and to make something of themselves. She also worked with me whenever I got sick and stayed home from school. She made learning fun and she was so passionate about her work that it made a significant impression on me.

Later on when my students would ask why I read things by holding them up close to my face, I would relate my personal story. I would tell them that we all faced challenges, and each of us had choices about how to respond. I had to adapt my work because of my vision, and I needed help to accomplish certain tasks, like grading papers. But I was doing something I loved, something I was passionate about. I was able to teach them and try to help them be successful in whatever they wanted to do in life. I helped shape their character and I wanted them to believe that a handicap does not have to hold you back.

While I enjoyed being a teacher, there was also a love in me for both medicine and the law. My family steered me away from these fields and encouraged me to enter the teaching profession. I think they were just trying to protect me from being disappointed. Down deep, however, I never gave up the idea of going to law school someday. I just kept it in the back of my mind.

Finding Dr. Price

One afternoon in 2003 I happened to be listening to the news on television, something I did not often do, when I heard an interview with an ophthalmologist in Indianapolis named Dr. Frank Price. He described a new FDA study involving a synthetic iris implant that reduced the amount of light entering the eyes. The next day I took a risk and called his office to see if I could possibly be a candidate for the study and got an appointment within a week.

He did many tests on my eyes and told me I would be a good candidate for the procedure. I was excited and optimistic. In the past, going to the eye doctor had always been a hassle. Dr. Price made it a different experience and was honest and open with me. I was equally impressed with his staff; they truly demonstrate the vision he has for his practice. They are professional, very friendly, really phenomenal in how they make patients feel that they are a person first, not a patient; an individual, not a number. They give that personal touch that means so much to all of us. I have always felt I can call with any questions I have and they will go out of their way to be sure I am satisfied and confident in their answers.

I think this is unusual. Many clinical practices are impersonal and make you feel rushed, rather than cared about. I think because Dr. Price is himself a humble man, the staff he attracts share his philosophy and that's what makes his practice thrive, along with his wonderful gifts as a surgeon, of course. His wife, Marianne, also complements him and shares his goal in making the Foundation well known and ultimately, one that helps as many people as possible. They do many different studies annually that benefit humanity, even those that don't pay any money, because they are passionate and committed to their work.

Iris Implant Surgery

What helped me go ahead with the surgery was a combination of curiosity ("Could this really be possible for me?") and the sense that Dr. Price could offer me a real option. With this surgery, I could move beyond acceptance of a life of dependence on others.

Dr. Price actually wanted to operate on my "best" eye first but I wanted my other eye done just in case the procedure didn't go as we planned. He agreed to my cautious strategy and I felt that he respected my feelings and showed compassion. A different doctor might have "overruled" my wishes and ignored my concerns, but not Dr. Price

During the 1.5-hour surgery, which was completely pain-free, Dr. Price frequently spoke to me. It was very comforting to hear his voice and his descriptions as the surgery progressed. I felt in safe hands. It was kind of like going on a great adventure. I was not heavily sedated, but I had this calm feeling the whole time.

The second day after surgery when they took the patch off my eye, I could see colors vividly and it was so great! I was actually able to see things so clearly that I had to blink in order to make myself believe what I was seeing. I was like a kid in a candy store: I wanted to see everything and I wanted to read something right away. It was wonderful. I asked for a mirror so I could see what my new green iris looked like, too!

The recovery period was straightforward; I received steroid eye drops to put into my eye three times a day to keep my body from rejecting the implant and to produce tears so my eye wouldn't get too dry. My recuperation consisted of an immediate one-week period in which my movements were restricted so as not to jar the transplant, but I was back in the water swimming competitively again in 8-12 weeks. I simply added a new pair of close fitting goggles to my attire in order to help adapt to the water. Dr. Price worked with me and I felt he was a great addition to my coaching team. Overall, the full healing took about a year; each day I got better and better.

How Life Has Changed

The implants have changed my life because I am able to do things I couldn't do before and never believed would be possible. Before the surgery, I could only see objects a few feet in front of me. Now I can see the world around me, and see it with crispness and clarity. I also wear glasses for reading and I am able to drive a car using a bioptic lens. This is a small lens attached to a pair of prescription glasses. When I lower my head, the lens gives me 20/20 vision so I can see distance.

The intent of the surgery was to help cut down the glare from the light coming into my eyes, but the implants have achieved something else: they have given my eyes a natural appearance. The whole experience has been a genuine "eye opener" for me.

It's not just *my* life, however, that's different. For my family and friends the surgery has been a life-changing event. They are all supportive and happy for me, of course, but they have had to adjust to my new independence. Especially my being able to drive a car – that makes them nervous. Eventually, we'll all get accustomed to my higher quality of life. I know they are as grateful as I am.

My life's work has changed, too. I really wanted to practice law; once my vision improved, I decided to go for it. I graduated from Indiana University Law School is 2005. I see the practice of law as a natural progression towards advocacy. The whole area of disabled rights interests me and I plan to do litigation work and be the voice for my disabled clients.

Advice to Readers

Keep an open mind and go out and be your own Number One advocate. You need to research the options that exist for your particular disability. The biggest thing is to be willing to take a risk once you find those options. If you don't, you will always have that nagging question, "What if I had done it?"

Whether it is a medical or other challenge, there are always adaptations that can be found to enable you to succeed. There's nothing you can't do if you are determined and willing to be flexible. Don't limit yourself.

My family and the core network of friends who have supported me throughout the years give me inspiration and courage. In difficult times, they have always encouraged me to overtake the obstacles placed in front of me. Whether it was medical or societal, their support and love helped me overcame those obstacles. I have great faith in my life and in my family. They provide me inner strength.

Sometimes people will say they'd like to change their lives, and there is almost always something we want to be different. Nobody's perfect. To learn something new every day and touch another person's life is so rewarding. It gives you strength and makes you a better person. You end up learning new things, too, that you might not have learned otherwise. To be an advocate for others has been a role I have enjoyed taking on and I look forward to doing it even more in my future work.

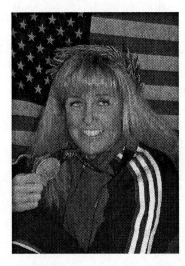

Trish Zorn

Note:

In 1948, Sir Ludwig Guttmann organized a sports competition involving World War II veterans with a spinal cord injury in Stoke Mandeville, England. Four years later, competitors from the Netherlands joined the games and an international movement was born. Olympic style games for athletes with a disability were organized for the first time in Rome in 1960, now called Paralympics. In Toronto in 1976, other disability groups were added and the idea of merging together different disability groups for international sport competitions was born. In the same year, the first Paralympic Winter Games took place in Sweden.

Today, the Paralympics are elite sport events for athletes from six different disability groups. They emphasize, however, the participants' athletic achievements rather than their disability. The movement has grown dramatically since its first days. The number of athletes participating in Summer Paralympic Games has increased from 400 athletes from 23 countries in Rome in 1960 to 3806 athletes from 136 countries in Athens in 2004.

The Paralympic Games have always been held in the same year as the Olympic Games. Since the Seoul 1988 Paralympic Games and the Albertville 1992 Winter Paralympic Games they have also taken place at the same venues as the Olympics. On 19 June 2001, an agreement was signed between IOC and IPC securing this practice for the future. From the 2012 bid process onwards, the host city chosen to host the Olympic Games will be obliged to also host the Paralympics.

Keratoconus

Ed Jagiela is a humorous, strong-willed man who shares a neat, trim home in Merrillville, Indiana with his wife, Joann, of 36 years. He has a ready laugh, and is clear about what matters most in life. In spite of the many challenges he has faced, Ed remains determined to live a life of joy, of gratitude and of service to others. We talked at his dining room table on a sunny day in September, the house filled with the fragrance of fresh-brewed coffee, potpourri and autumn flowers.

The world was always a blurry place for me. I just took it for granted and assumed that's the way it was supposed to be. By the time I was in the fourth grade, I wore glasses. It was extremely difficult for me to accommodate to the classroom because most of the time I couldn't see what was on the blackboard. My grades suffered and each successive pair of glasses helped, but the lenses just kept getting thicker and thicker as my eyesight worsened.

I was also a sickly child and had many allergies growing up. Other kids teased me and I learned to walk away from fights and acquired "street smarts" in order to survive. I learned never to turn my back on anyone because I had no big brother to back me up. I had only myself. Looking back, I know I developed an attitude problem; I was not Mr. Nice.

My parents were good-hearted people but they were part of the Depression generation. You didn't waste things and you didn't expect to be given things. You didn't cry and you didn't lean on others. You learned to rely on yourself and you learned not to ask others for help. Independence was the most important thing my parents instilled in me. I recall that whenever I asked to go and do something as a child, their standard response was that if I couldn't walk, take the bus or ride my bike there, I just couldn't go. They would not coddle me in any way and it made me very strong. I learned not to depend on them for a lot of extra help; they emphasized that I had to do things for myself.

When I met Joann, my future wife, in high school I had a fierce independent streak and I didn't trust many people. She gradually influenced me to begin to soften that attitude. We went steady for a few years and then got married in 1969. I was only making about $60 a week as a meat cutter at the time. Working as a meat cutter and being visually impaired was definitely challenging and I had a lot of small accidents in the beginning. Once I actually got a knife stuck in my leg; I just put a tourniquet around it and drove myself to a hospital.

Joann worked in an ophthalmologist's office during those years, and I got my first contact lenses from her doctor when I was in my late twenties, along with a diagnosis of keratoconus. This is a condition in which the cornea gradually thins and bulges. Normal eyes are round; mine are cone-shaped. I also had astigmatism and was told it would get progressively worse. I was given hard contact lenses but they were bad for me because they were rigid and often fell out. I tried soft ones and liked them better. I remember driving home with my wife the first day I got them and asking her to stop the car and pull over. She was concerned and asked me what was wrong. I told her it was the first time I had seen clouds with texture; up to that point they were just white objects in the sky. It was an incredible experience.

By the time I went to work at the Ford Motor Company at age 36, I had given up on contact lens and gone back to wearing glasses. Even with specially fitted glasses, I could only see a small hazy amount. As before, I learned to accommodate to a new work routine and new duties. After awhile I knew my way around the work area so well I could have done the job blindfolded. I let my wife drive me to work until I learned the way and then from that point on, I drove myself. It never mattered if it was dark, sunny or snowy. I learned to recognize objects along the road and certain landmarks so I could gauge distance and I learned how to get back and forth from my home to the plant.

During those years, I had a routine: I would work 12 hours a day, come home, take a shower and then go to the kids' activities. My two daughters, Jennifer and Diane, were so important to my wife and I. Everything we did was for them. They were in cheerleading, tap and jazz. Like parents everywhere, I would often feel so tired that my mind would say "no" but my mouth always said "yes."

I didn't think of my vision as a major obstacle during these years because I was able to get my driver's license. I learned to squint my eyes when taking the driving vision test until I could see the letters well enough to pass the test. I am not sure I would have passed me, but I was glad that *they* did because it gave me a lot of freedom.

One Crisis and then Another

I woke up one morning in August 1996 and my left eye had started turning green. When I got to my doctor's office he immediately sent me to Indianapolis to meet with Dr. Price. By the time I got there I could not see out of either eye and I was in a great deal of pain. I met Dr. Price in the emergency room, and started receiving infection medicine in each eye. Within a short time, we signed the consent for surgery and my left eye was removed due to the severity of the infection, and was replaced with a prosthesis. Day by day it was "iffy." It took two weeks of care and reconstruction before I could be discharged. Oddly enough, there had been another man admitted with the same kind of infection during my stay and that man died, so I was very fortunate to survive.

My first impression of Dr. Price was that he was a godsend; he worked on me and helped me so much that if he ever moves away, I will follow him because I don't trust anybody else. He is someone who gives information to me straight; he never tries to water things down. I need that kind of approach and appreciate it. He is calm, collected, a man who knows what he's doing with very clear goals. He has a great backup, too, in his wife Marianne; she is really great. They are both so dedicated.

As my keratoconus advanced, I twice developed a serious condition, acute corneal hydrops, which occurs when the Descemet's membrane ruptures and causes corneal edema, or swelling. In some cases, the hydrops may resolve itself, as it did with me the first time it happened. However, the second time, only three weeks before Christmas in 2000, I became blind. I remember waking up at home that morning thinking it was still night and then realizing that I could not see. I found my way to my neighbor's home and asked him to call Joann. She came home immediately and once more, we headed off with fear and anxieties to Indianapolis to meet with Dr. Price.

He told me then, "it is time for a transplant," and I believed every word. He also told me that there was only a 20% chance that the transplant would succeed because of the heavily scarred sclera and cornea.

Four months later, on April 12, 2001, I received my corneal transplant and it worked! I was in and out in three hours. My eye was heavily bandaged and the next day when they took them off, I could see the big E on the eye chart! What a thrill! Dr. Price was beaming and happy, of course. It was a miracle really and there was not a dry eye in his office that day. He is so darn good at what he does. He is not someone who would ever give up on you. I have a deep heartfelt respect for him and he's never steered me wrong.

Life Lessons

When you are blind, you learn to compensate and trust your other senses. There is no color in that world; it is all black and white. I have tried to put into my memory banks the colors of happy memories; especially those made with my two kids. For example, I used to come home after working 12 hours when my girls were in school, and one of them would have left a note for me on the steps saying, "I made it in cheerleading!" or things like that. Years later I got to walk each of them down the aisle on their wedding day. Each of these moments were so moving for all of us because there had been times when we had wondered if I would ever get to do that special Dad's task. God allowed it to happen and I am so grateful.

Life is too short to wish it away; do what you want to do now because you don't want to be sorry later on and have regrets. When I give talks, it's hard saying that to some of the people in the audience who may be feeling sorry for themselves. That emotion doesn't work for me; I can only feel sorry for myself so long. I end up laughing at myself most of the time.

Being married to Joann, the greatest woman in the world, is a joy. She keeps me on my toes and keeps me going. She and my two beautiful daughters are my inspiration, although they say that *I* inspire *them*.

God has given me new goals in my life since my disability. I love being able to serve other people through the Lions Club and the Eye Bank. Dawn Hill is someone who has helped get me on the right road. I was slipping into depression when she came along and got me out speaking. It has made a huge difference in my life and opened up a whole new world to me. I am committed to helping others to believe that they have the ability to go beyond a disability.

Having vision difficulties throughout my life has changed me and made me a fuller person. I have a greater appreciation for the beauty of this world. I love seeing the Harvest Moon, seeing the leaves change and seeing the sun when I get up in the morning. I love snowflakes and how each one is unique. Life is truly a great adventure.

I am more emotional now than I've ever been. I was taught that men don't cry; well, stuff happens and your emotions come out. I used to be quite a grumpy person, even hard to get along with, some would say, but being blind and then recovering my sight has changed me. I am also getting older, and that has caused me to reflect on my life and softened me, too.

I continue to face physical challenges. Right now, I anticipate having more surgery in the next few months, not for my vision, but for my back. I have a pinched nerve up high and it will require inserting a titanium plate and screws. (I asked the doctors to be sure and place the screws on each side of my neck so I can be Frankenstein at Halloween!) But I also plan on going to Italy with Joann on a cruise next spring and I don't intend to let back surgery interfere with that.

Advice to Readers

(1) I think the best way to deal with any illness is to become educated about it; learn as much as you can by reading and talking to others who face the same condition as you do. The Internet is a great source of support and information.

(2) Make sure you have a great doctor, one you trust and have confidence in, so you can feel like you're partners and allies.

(3) Talk to your family members and make sure they know the facts, too. That will help them feel stronger and better able to cope with the changes that will be inevitable.

(4) Go with your feelings and trust your gut, but don't slide into depression; look at what God has given you in this loss and count your blessings. There is always someone worse off than you.

(5) Make your life your own interesting movie; be the

director, the producer and the star. Create the happy ending you want. Inspire others and be grateful for the closeness of your family and friends.

(6) Take a few chances in life and go for the gold. Don't just sit back and let somebody else make decisions for you.

(7) Keep going and keep your sense of humor. There are a thousand answers for every challenge you face; it's up to you to decide which choice you want to make.

Corneal Transplants

"The Good Lord Sitting on His Shoulder"

Bob Higginbotham lives in Pawtucket, Rhode Island and his speech has a characteristic New England accent that is readily recognizable. A successful businessman, Bob was forced to retire early because of a visual impairment that worsened over time. It was his vital and enduring faith in God, his desperation and a fortunate set of circumstances that combined to offer him a "second chance" at the age of 78. Deeply spiritual, Bob has a sense that his sight was restored because God has something more for him to accomplish before he leaves this earth.

I was born with a cataract in my left eye; as I grew older, it calcified in my left pupil and became a bright white dot that took away much of my sight. In grade school, other kids called me "polka dot eye." Fortunately, my right eye was perfect; the only thing I suffered from was diminished depth perception. For example, when I played center field on a baseball team, I wouldn't know if the ball coming toward me was a "pop up" or over my head.

By the time I was 68 years old, the vision in my right eye had deteriorated. My ophthalmologist was concerned about me after removing a cataract. The vision did not come back fully and the edema worsened. I then went to a specialist, Dr. Chou, who asked me to consider a corneal transplant. It was a tough decision to make, knowing full well that I was already blind in my left eye. The prospect of being without any sight for 8 to 12 months while the transplant healed left me cold.

Then, Dr. Chou went to a symposium and heard Dr. Frank Price speak about a new cornea-sparing transplant he was offering in his practice. She told me later that she immediately thought of me when she heard him describe one of its advantages over traditional transplants: a much quicker healing period. She is a highly capable doctor and I trusted her recommendation that I make an appointment with Dr. Price, but I have to admit I was a bit leery at first. After all, no one in the entire New England region was doing this surgery, and at age 78, I was cautious.

My biggest concern about a traditional corneal transplant was that I'd be forced to be a couch potato for 9 to 12 months until my vision was restored, and I was afraid that this level of inactivity would result in other ailments developing. I prayed for guidance and weighed my options. If I did nothing, I would lose my driver's license and being without a car would be tough. I was actually feeling pretty desperate and this new surgery certainly had a great appeal. I discussed it at length with my beautiful wife, Dorothy, and decided to fly to Indianapolis for the consultation.

A Happy Office

When I met Dr. Price and his team I couldn't believe what I experienced. I've been a clinical lab owner and visited many practices over the years so I know something about customer service. Each person on his staff treated me with respect and there was an atmosphere I can only describe as "happy" in his offices. And he's got to be famous, he's so talented, yet I found Dr. Price to be completely down to earth. I was thrilled to death! It went a long way toward making me lose my concerns and replacing them with confidence.

My wife and I decided that I should go ahead with the surgery and I actually had some fun in the operating room. In fact, Dorothy was waiting for me outside the surgery area and she asked me later on, "What was going on in there? I could hear you laughing!" I had told a story to the operating team and the punchline was the phrase "Baby cakes." Well, when I was being wheeled out of the surgical suite, the staff lined up and in unison, said, "Bye, bye Baby Cakes!" It was a very, very pleasant experience.

I spent two weeks in Indianapolis and came back for checkups with Dr. Price before finally being given permission to fly home to Rhode Island. I will never forget this one instance that showed me Dr. Price's true caring as a doctor. It was two days after surgery and he saw something in my eye he didn't like. He actually came in that Sunday and opened the practice just to work on my eye again. And he was so kind about it! The transplant still was a bit iffy and he fixed the problem. Imagine! Coming in on a Sunday to see a patient; I will never forget it.

Within six weeks after surgery I was seeing better than I had in 30 years! In fact, I am still waiting for glasses because each time I go in to my doctor's office, my eyesight has gotten better.

A New Lease on Life

My life has changed so much since the transplant. It has given my wife and I both a new lease on life. I have been a volunteer in a hospice but had taken a leave because I could no longer drive. Just recently I have been able to get back into it again. And I can play golf now and actually see the ball. I go to Mass each morning and it feels so good to be able to do that again. My son and daughter run my business for me, but now, if they needed me to, I could help out. I am an active, productive member of society again. I can do what I want and I am independent once more.

My restored sight has impacted everyone in my close-knit family. I have six children: John is the oldest and teaches medical terminology at a local college; Tommy is in the security field; Ken is the son who runs my business along with Ann, my daughter; another daughter, Susan, is a housewife and Julie is a schoolteacher. I am very proud of each of them and they have given us a lot of joy. My wife, Dorothy, is a sweetie; she is a wonderful woman and a supportive partner. She has always been there for me. For example, when I went into business for myself we had six kids still at home. I was 48 years old and it was a big gamble because I had never owned a company before. She sat me down one night at the kitchen table, and said, "You've got to do this because if you don't you'll end up a miserable old man. And I don't want to live with a miserable old man." That was just the message I needed to hear and we went ahead with our gamble. It turned out well and it is still a successful company today.

I think one of the biggest changes for me since the surgery is connected to my life purpose. I had been going along doing my best, but now I feel strongly that God had a reason for saving my sight, and there is something He wants me yet to do. I have never had this feeling before. It's very strong and I can sense it when I pray or during quiet moments. You know some people determine their vocation early in their lives; for others, it happens much later. I think I am one of those. I plan to keep praying each day, and listening for God's guidance.

Advice to Readers

I have lived a long time and I have made my share of mistakes. I believe strongly in my faith. I prayed a lot before deciding to have the surgery, but at the same time, I think you have to be philosophical about life and accept whatever happens. The good Lord gave me the feeling that I should go ahead with the surgery; He guided me each step of the way. So I would recommend prayer, along with finding out the facts about your situation and taking the input of professionals you respect as you decide what to do.

I believe in being a good steward in life. Saint Francis of Assisi is someone I have always admired and found inspiring. When he was given clothing, for example, he only kept it until he found someone else who needed it more than he did. He felt that the material things he was given were only his for a time; that he was keeping in trust the resources that all came from God. Dr. Price, who's also named Francis, has been given tremendous gifts and he can produce what I call "miracles" for others through the use of those talents. He gives people a chance for a new life and that is miraculous in itself.

If I could talk directly with the readers of this book, I would encourage them to seek out Dr. Price; if he can work a miracle, he will. You'll never be sorry you went to him for help. Look into your heart and if you need a miracle – that may not be the right word, but it is the one I choose - there is no better place to go. And no better man than Dr. Price.

Postscript: Bob wrote a letter to Dr. Price a few weeks after his surgery and before he knew that he'd be interviewed in this book. The letter was circulated among clinic staff and touched many hearts with its authentic and heartfelt emotion. It is reprinted here as it was received:

Dear Dr. Price,

Just a short note to let you know how I am coming along. I know that Dr. Chou has been in touch with you, but I wanted to talk to you personally.

First of all, at the present time I am seeing, after only six weeks, better than I have in at least fifteen years. Last week, my sight checked in at 20/30 and it's getting better all the time.

How do I say "thank you" to you? You took an old man who was on the verge of being severely handicapped for the rest of his life and made him feel young again and enabled him to remain active for the rest of his life. What you did for me you did for many other people as well because it affected my wife, my children, my grandchildren and maybe some others that I may be able to help, in the future, because of you.

Your skill, kindness, consideration and caring, I will never forget. I will always remember you and, in remembering, keep you in my prayers.

You must be very proud also of your staff; every one of them treated me with much kindness. Remember me to them and give my regards. By the way the staff in surgery was also great to me. Tell them, please, that "Baby Cakes" says "Thank you" and sends his regards. They will know!

I pray the good Lord will keep you healthy and able to do for others what you did for me. Thanks again.

Love,

Bob Higginbotham

Corneal Transplants

"Becoming More Than You Are"

It's hard to think of a more inspiring figure than Donald Lane; his quiet way of speaking is in harmony with his quiet manner of relating to others. A warm and gentle man, he has been humbled by serious life challenges that began at birth. Having once been blind, he is deeply appreciative of the beauty of Nature, and the capacity for hope that lies within all of us. He and his wife, Sue, also visually impaired, are a remarkable couple whose love and courage bring a healing example to the world.

My visual impairment is the result of birth defects when I was born; the doctors theorize that my Mom had German measles. She probably didn't even notice because she already had three children in diapers at that point! I was born with glaucoma, a misplaced pupil in one eye and three holes in the iris of my other eye.

As I became an adult, I was able to see well out of the eye that had a single pupil and my vision was 20/40. The only accommodation I had to make was to drive only during the day and to use special outside rearview mirrors. Then in 1976, when I went to renew my drivers' license, I was unable to pass the vision test. I knew then that I was going to face more serious problems with my sight. At that time, my doctor did not know exactly what was wrong. Three years earlier, he had suggested that I go to St. Louis to have surgery to restore my vision. I did so and my vision returned. Two years later, I had to have my first corneal transplant because the iris closed up in my good eye and I was unable to see. The surgery involved cutting a little hole in it to allow the light to get through.

In 1981, I had another corneal transplant that worked for three years and then failed. Two years later, I underwent a third transplant and by then, I had also developed cataracts in my left eye, my "good eye." That cornea transplant never did clear up my vision. I came back to Indianapolis to see Dr. David Kenney, my regular doctor and a wonderful man. He suggested that I see Dr. Price. It was 1984 when Dr. Price performed my fourth cornea transplant and my vision was once again restored to me.

Meeting Dr. Price

When I first met Dr. Price and his team they seemed technically advanced. He was ready for any problem my eyes had to offer; he seemed to be anxious to make things right to help me see better. He was kind and I liked the people he had working for him. It said a lot about him as much as anything else did. They were an exceptionally kind and competent staff.

Since I had already undergone several successful surgeries, I never felt "on the fence" as some others might have been about having yet another eye surgery. In addition, some family members had successfully undergone minor surgeries, so I generally had confidence in the medical profession. Talking to Dr. Price was key, though; he had a good logical explanation of what to do and how it would help. More than anything, people have to think logically and see what sounds reasonable when making a major decision such as eye surgery.

Dr. Price is a reassuring doctor; he is very kind and it shows in everything he does. He must have a lot of strength and stamina, too, because his job has to be difficult but he never seems exhausted or irritable. He works late and on weekends and at all hours and yet he's always patient.

Facing Life's Challenges

The thing that amazes me today is the tiny amount of pain that is involved in a corneal transplant. I have had a number of surgeries in the past, and things have improved so much. An example is my 2003 recuperation: it was fairly short and in just a few days, I noticed a big improvement. I had surgery on June 19th after being virtually blind for twelve years and, on that July 4th, I went outside and saw the sunset for the first time. It was awesome.

One thing that people should be mindful of and that's their first month after surgery. It's very important to take care of your wound and your incision. Do everything your doctor tell you. That's the core of it. Don't lift anything heavier than a milk carton for the first month. For the next month, don't lift over 20 pounds; then for six months, don't lift anything over 50 pounds. Don't get your eye wet for the first two weeks and use an eye shield for two months. Wear glasses during the day so you limit the risk of injury to your eye. These are small burdens to put up with in exchange for receiving improved vision.

I have worn correction glasses since my surgery in 2003. My wife, Sue, is also visually impaired and she uses a device called a CC-TV (closed circuit TV). It's a TV mounted on a stand with a camera underneath it that points down. There's a table under the camera that allows you to place objects on it, like a newspaper, and the camera magnifies the images and shows them on the TV screen so you can read it. I tried using it when I first lost my vision but was never successful.

After the surgery in 2003, however, I learned to use it to read. I cannot read for long because it takes a lot of concentration, but I can use it to look up the prescription number on a little bottle, for example. It's a great aid to my daily life.

We are facing some health challenges in our family right now. My wife's kidneys have failed and she goes by bus for dialysis three days a week and uses a wheelchair. When she returns from dialysis, I help by waiting for the bus to come and then I go out and get her inside. It's a great feeling to be useful. I also help by putting her pills in her pill tray. The visiting nurse has been coming because Sue has had a wound on her foot, but that's healed up so I will soon be back to doing that for her. I also Braille her medicine bottles for her.

Sue was a medical transcriptionist before she became ill but she's stuck in her wheelchair right now and has not worked for two years. I used to be an electronics engineer and I retired in 1995. I like to tinker around the house, but too often when I take things apart, I cannot get them back together again! Sue gets a little frustrated with me on those occasions. Luckily, I know a few people I can call to come over and help me out when I've gotten myself in a jam like that!

Greatest Life Lessons Learned

I think life presents all of us with difficulties and we can choose to look at them as something that stops our progress, or as obstacles we have to meet and overcome. If you wish to grow and become more than you are, you *have* to overcome obstacles. It requires a combination of things: the most important is a belief in yourself, and a willingness to work at facing your fears and getting outside your comfort level. The best thing you can do is to believe in God.

For a long time, I didn't have a great belief in God. I didn't see Him in my personal daily life and during that period, I searched high and low for the meaning of life. I was trying to find myself. Little by little, I began to see things that were unexplainable and didn't make sense. It was then that I realized God was in my life to give me strength, and to make up for my shortcomings. He blesses me far more than I deserve - I don't know how else to say it. I read a beautiful book called *Return to Love* by Marianne Williamson, and that's what brought it all together for me.

My wife Sue is a great inspiration and a gift to me. I met her in 1994 when she was in an unhappy marriage. We were in a breakfast group called the "Blind Breakfast Bunch" started by Terry, a friend of mine who was blind and on dialysis. He had undergone a kidney transplant and ended up with all this time on his hands and became bored. So he called up a few friends and went out to eat; that group just grew and grew. Terry died 7 years ago but the group continues to grow and meet on a regular basis. It's a legacy of his love.

Sue was one of those people in the group who was always bright and cheerful. She never had a negative thing to say and I always liked talking to her. She divorced her husband in 1998 and we began dating the following year. She had breast cancer that same year and one day she told me that she was finishing up her radiation and I said, "Well we should celebrate that." I asked her out for lunch, she said yes, and we just fell in love with each other. We were married two years ago. She is the bright star in my life; she chases my loneliness away and inspires me to do things. She is the reason I get up in the morning and go to bed at night. We were meant to be together.

Advice to Readers

Have faith; try to make your life better by using the tools available to reach out to other people. Give something of your time, energy or talents to help others. Try to find out as much as you can because you cannot make a good decision unless you have information. And don't give up.

Once, briefly, I was tempted to give up. I had had problems with my eyes for many years, but I really didn't have what I think of as "true" blindness. Then, in 1991, my real challenge came when I had a detached retina in my left eye. I underwent two surgeries that failed; I was off work four weeks with the first attempt. Hand motions at six inches were all I could see. I was blind.

It was extremely hard to face going back to work like that, and it was a real low point in my life. But I did go back; I had a

91

friend take me shopping and I bought a white cane. I just said to myself, "I can't stop here." I called my boss and announced "I am coming back" and he responded "Ok." They found a way to use me and I kept telling myself, "They didn't hire me for my eyes; they hired me for my brain."

Four years later, I retired because it was the best thing to do. I did not retire because of my eyes, but for other reasons. I saw people over the age of 50 who were being let go so the company could hire younger workers for less money. They also moved work overseas for cheaper labor. It was a tough labor market and I knew it was time for me to leave.

This experience taught me that being able to reinvent yourself is what is required of workers today. I was 48 years old when I retired and a neighbor came over and said, "You are too young to sit around and do nothing." But I managed to do exactly that for a year. Then, on the very same day, I got two calls; one from an engineering consulting firm to go back to work, and the other was from an agency wanting me to volunteer. I accepted both, and worked as a contract consultant for awhile and committed time to volunteering, which I still do each week. I tutor people in math for their GED and occasionally work in the computer lab to help people read and write Braille. It's rewarding to see people change and grow who have been through the same difficulties I have.

It's so touching to see people change from the first day I meet them and they tell me their story. Often, they see their life as really bad; their wife may have left them, they may have lost their job and they might not be allowed to see their kids anymore. Then six months later I meet them on the bus one morning and they are going to college to learn a new set of skills. It makes me weep. I feel so blessed to have had a hand in their growth and to know that I've made a small difference in their life.

Giving of yourself helps you put your own challenges in perspective, and is something to be grateful for each and every day. We are able to heal ourselves as we help heal others. It's another one of God's daily miracles to appreciate.

Corneal Transplants

"Give Me a Blue One!"

Pastor Clarence Moore has a warm and ready smile that immediately put me at ease when we met in his comfortable office at the Northside New Era Baptist Church. His lifework is an inner city ministry that he relishes as his life's calling. A humorous man, Pastor Moore enjoys speaking in a playful manner to elicit shared laughter. Equally eloquent at other times, he inspires listeners to strive to find their life purpose in order to serve the world and to serve God.

My vision challenges began when I was in my early twenties and working at General Motors in the purchasing department. One day a co-worker came to my cubicle and said, "Clarence, do you realize how close you are holding that paper to your face?" It dawned on me then that I had gradually adjusted to a significant loss of sight and it shocked me to learn how much accommodation I had made just to carry out my work. Not long after, an incident happened in a softball game that was equally sobering. A normal ground ball came towards me and hit me right in the forehead. My wife asked me later, "How did you let that happen? Did you not see that ball?" I had to admit to her that my eyesight was diminishing. I had not fully realized it myself until then. I should also mention that my Mother has been legally blind all her life. She had two detached retinas and, when I admitted my failing sight, I wasn't sure but that I might be headed down that same road.

At the time I was supervising a good Christian lady who wore thick Coke-bottle glasses. Peggy and I became good friends and one day she came to work without her glasses and I was startled. I asked her where they were and how was she able to see without them. She said, "Oh, I have to tell you about the miracle. I had laser surgery with a young doctor in Indianapolis named Dr. Francis Price." I had never heard of laser surgery and she was so enthusiastic that it made a strong impression on me. Being free of those thick glasses made a positive difference in her self-confidence and her appearance.

Time to Get Help

I couldn't see well enough to drive at night although it was hard to admit it. One frightful night, I picked up my two small children from the babysitter and I simply could not get home. I could not turn left or right or read the road signs. I still remember vividly how frightening that night was. I had to stop and call my wife to tell her what was happening. I made it home, finally, but only because God was looking out for us. On another occasion, I drove some friends home and hit two or three mailboxes on the way and scared us half to death.

A few years later I accepted my calling into the ministry. By then, I was seeing so badly I could not drive myself to seminary classes and so my wife had to provide transportation. My eyesight was very blurry, and I had to enlarge things in print in order to be able to read them so I studied by listening to my wife read chapters to me. She would read and then tell me what she thought were the key points and we would discuss them. You know, even to this day, when I see colleagues I went to school with they give credit to my wife, Hope, for my A's in seminary. They would overhear her talking to me in the halls between classes and they thought she was my "secret weapon" for academic success. In keeping with her character, she always defended me by pointing out that I had a great memory and that's how I got such good grades.

When I graduated seminary and became a minister, I could not see my Bible or my sermon notes. I couldn't go back and forth between the two to find the right phrases as I preached. As a result, I was very limited and ineffective; good, passionate preaching requires the ability to stay in the flow as you inspire people. I felt my limitations were not what God wanted. There had to be a better way and I decided that it was time to do something about my sight.

My optometrist had treated me for keratoconus and astigmatism and referred me to an ophthalmologist in Kokomo, Indiana so I started there. After the exam, I told him I wanted a second opinion and I asked him to recommend someone. He responded that he'd like to handle my condition himself and told me that I needed a corneal transplant. After he explained that he had just started doing these procedures, I thought it over and got a referral from him. It was Dr. Francis W. Price, Jr. in Indianapolis.

Probabilities in my Favor

I came to Indianapolis to meet Dr. Price. He was a young man around my own age but he seemed very knowledgeable and he had experience with all kinds of things that impacted the cornea. I wanted to put the probabilities in my favor; I thought my chances of improvement were better with Dr. Price even though having his care and surgery would mean traveling to Indianapolis.

Dr. Price was an impressive doctor. He first tried hard contact lenses on me for about three months but I couldn't wear them. He explained how the football shape of my eye differed from the baseball shape of a normal eye. The lenses irritated my eyes and he said, "Well, we have no other choice but this transplant procedure." I was scared to death, of course, but I knew that he was skillful. His communication of my condition to my wife and me was outstanding. I was encouraged by his prognosis. The other thing that impressed me was sitting in the lobby and realizing how many people came from all over the Midwest to see him. I had this thought, "All these people can't be wrong." Especially my friend Peggy who was so high on Dr. Price; I had great trust in her judgement.

I remember an early conversation between Dr. Price and I about the transplant; he said to me, "We are going to get you the best cornea in the world." I jokingly replied, "Well if I have to have a new cornea, make sure it's blue." He looked at me funny and asked, "Excuse me?" I did not know then that corneas are clear without any color, and so I explained further, "Well if you have blue eyes, you get promoted. I may have the wrong color skin, but with blue eyes, I might have half a chance of getting promoted." At that, we both laughed together but he had the last word and said, "Well I can't help you with a blue one; you're stuck with brown eyes!"

It was the year 2000 and I had my left cornea, my "worst" eye, replaced with a transplant. During surgery, I was put to sleep and when I woke up, I had no pain in my eye at all. One admonition I remembering receiving before being discharged was not to sneeze and I can remember feeling I wanted to sneeze so badly, but I would not let it happen. (It is hard to hold back a sneeze for hours, I can tell you!) Twenty-four hours later, Dr. Price took my bandages off. I looked at him with awe and said, "Wow, I can see you really well." I know that God used him to work a miracle. He had changed my world, but he didn't want any accolades. I was ready to shout it from the rooftops but he was calm and just patted me on the shoulder, saying, "You did well."

When I got home that day, I could see my dear little children's' faces just as clearly as I had seen Dr. Price and it was a moment I will never forget. It makes me emotional even now just remembering it. And I could also see my lovely wife's face clearly, too. What gifts from God!

My recuperation took 3-4 months and I was off work during that whole time. I had been assigned to work in a chemical area and I really didn't want to be in that environment while I was healing. Neither Dr. Price nor I thought it a good idea for me to return to work under those circumstances. I also could not do any heavy lifting or even bend over to tie my shoes. Other than that, I just rested and took life a bit more slowly than usual. When it was over, I was able to drive again, even at night, and I had no more blurriness. I could enjoy reading stories to my children. I could go to soccer games and actually see my child score, rather than just hear about it from another parent seated nearby.

In 2004, I had a corneal transplant in my right eye. Dr. Price predicted that it would do better than my first transplant because, in the interim, he had gained even more experience and the technology had gotten better. My left eye had become my dominant eye and the right eye had become dependent. With correction in both eyes my overall vision would be much better. Dr. Price did two relaxing incisions after the transplant to improve my vision as much as possible and I had LASIK twice. My vision became 20/30 – another of God's miracles.

How Life Has Changed

The miracle of sight allows this preacher to "...rightly divide the word of Truth..." as I preach the Gospel. The sight that has come through the hands of Dr. Price allows me to not just function as an average pastor, but my sightedness has allowed me to use *all* of my gifts with greater confidence. I owe my ministerial work to him and his staff. God used each of them to bring miracles into our lives.

I have been able to take a trip to Africa with my family, for example, and I was able to see all the sights and experience the people, the land, etc. I was able to travel to Greece this summer, too, and all of these things have come because I have been given the miracle of being in Dr. Price's care. He has literally opened the world up to me.

My children are now grown; Curtis is the oldest and he's at medical school, Courtney is a teacher and Cristen is a writer. I am proud of them and sharing life with them as a sighted parent is one of the many "residual blessings" God has given me with my sight.

I believe Dr. Price's work goes far beyond him, and I hope he realizes this. God is using him to touch lives and work miracles. In essence, Dr. Price is actually giving a new life to each of his patients and there's no way of gauging how far that life reaches and how many other lives will be impacted.

Life Lessons

I think God used vision failure as a tool to reorder my steps. I had been active in my church but I didn't have ministry on my mind. He used my lack of sight to really talk with me and get my attention. There's a similar story in the Bible about Paul on the Damascus Road who was blind. God sent Annais to uncover the scales from Paul's eyes and restore his sight. I don't think I would have heard God call me to a higher mission if I had not been losing my sight. And He could have left me in that state but then Peggy walked into my office that day without glasses and I saw that look on her face and I witnessed a new life emerging.

Each day when I wake up I am reminded of the fact that I could lose my sight again if these corneas are rejected. That knowledge continually gives me the sense of being in the presence of God. I have empathy for drug abusers and alcoholics that I work with in my ministry. I have a sense of their struggles as I sit across from them. Not that I struggle with my sight every day but I know the potential is there to lose it, just as they can lose their sobriety. In that sense, we are sharing a journey of gratitude.

Advice to Readers

There is, indeed, help for those who struggle with sight issues. Someone like Dr. Price and his organization are worth a visit or a consultation. I have noticed one thing about him: he has incredible patience. He's not in this for the money because he takes so much time with his patients; he does not just run into the exam room and rush you into surgery. He spends time getting to know his patients. There were days when I felt impatient and wanted him to go faster, but he would just take his time to find the best care possible for me. Readers should try and find someone like this when they are seeking a doctor to help with vision problems.

In closing, I would tell readers that the accounts you are reading are of real and normal people whose quality of life has been enhanced immensely as the result of taking a worthwhile risk. Have courage and have faith in God as you go forward to find the best care for your eyes.

Laser Refractive Surgery

"Liberation"

I met Chris Wright at the Broad Ripple Starbucks where I interviewed him as we sat in front of a warm fireplace on a rainy winter day in Indianapolis. Dressed fashionably in a pink shirt with complementary tie, cowboy boots and a dark blue suit, Chris was easygoing and friendly. He is a familiar figure to local residents who watch him describe the weather each evening on television. Trained as a meteorologist, his on-camera demeanor is relaxed and quick-witted, the same as his responses during our interview. It's clear that Chris is comfortable with himself, and enjoys life with a sense of adventure.

I started wearing glasses when I was nine years old. Before I got them, I always had to sit at the front of the class so I could see the board. Other kids teased me constantly and that made me feel shy and different. Even though I was a smart kid, the teachers noticed that I was having trouble reading and so I had an eye test. Sure enough, I needed to wear glasses. In those days, glasses were not very stylish, so I had to wear these big horn-rimmed ones for years. Here I was this skinny kid, wearing thick glasses, smart and not very athletic - it was like always wearing a sign that said, "Kick me!"

When contact lenses were introduced, I started wearing them to get away from those awful glasses. The expense associated with wearing contacts was one of the things that made me decide to have laser surgery. The thin ones tore all the time and I was always buying replacements. Then there was a law passed that said you had to get an eye exam each time you got new contacts. The time and money it took just did not make any sense and I wanted to simplify my life. Plus my vision was getting a little bit worse and I was ready to find a solution that would last.

I was working at a local station and heard some commercials about Dr. Price doing laser surgery. When I first heard how quick a procedure it was, that was a plus and then when I compared all of the expenses of money and time associated with wearing contacts, the exams, the solution, etc, it looked like a really good investment. I called and got more information about the procedure and the costs, and made an appointment to meet Dr. Price.

I liked him immediately and felt comfortable with him. That was really important to me. Having eye surgery is not like someone putting a bandage on an "owie" as my daughter says. It's serious business; if it goes wrong, it's catastrophic. I wanted to be sure that he was someone I could trust. Just talking to him, he never made me feel like he was rushed. He was the actually second doctor I had spoken to about laser surgery. The first one just seemed in too big a hurry. I did not have a good feeling about him and I sure didn't want him rushing in to do my eye surgery.

I did not want a quick fix, but I wanted a solution that would last. Dr Price took the time to put me at ease; he was calm and very knowledgeable. He answered all my questions and by the time I left that day, I felt informed. He showed me how my vision would change using a computer program that I thought was pretty cool. They educated me enough to feel sure that this was what I wanted to do. I left without any doubts that this was the best solution for me.

One week later I returned to have the surgery. There was no special prep for it, other than I was told not to wear contacts for 24 hours before having the procedure, and to have someone drive me home. I made arrangements to have a friend of mine drop me off that morning and drive me home later. (I was off work, of course, and took full advantage of it by just going home and going to bed after the surgery was finished.)

I remember walking down the hall toward the waiting room, and being unable to read any of the posters or articles on the wall because I wasn't wearing my contacts or glasses. I got to the room and joined a group of people all waiting to go into surgery. The nurses gave us each a pill to relax and as we sat there, they explained what they needed us to do once the laser surgery began which wasn't much: we just had to look at the red light and not move our eyes. That sounded simple enough to me and I was eager to get it done.

I got into the surgery room, laid on the bed and was told to focus on the red light and they reminded me not to move my head or my eyes. Once the procedure began, there was no sensation of pain, or discomfort of any kind. But no one had told me that I would smell a slight burning odor. It was kind of funny really because I was lying there telling myself, 'Dude, I can smell fire but no one else seems alarmed. Don't move, just relax. I am just lying here quietly and they are all being so calm, it must be fine.' I could hear the laser going tick, tick, tick, tick. Then it was over and they began working on the other eye. It seemed like it was about twenty minute's total time that passed and then they were done.

They had tested my eyes and while I had been 20/200 one eye and 20/400 in the other prior to surgery, when they re-tested, my eyes were 20/10 right then and there. As I walked back down that same hall, I could actually see the photos clearly and read the articles I couldn't just minutes before. It was just that quick and just that remarkable.

They were doing a study at the time and I ended up having both of my eyes done at once, but there were other people who only had one eye done on that day. I have a philosophy about being part of clinical studies. I know as a scientist myself that progress is made through what is learned in studies. I would encourage anyone who has a chance to be part of a study not to feel afraid, but to consider it an opportunity to help advance scientific knowledge.

At the time of my laser surgery, I was working at one of the local stations and they actually did a story on me having surgery; they told the "before and after" story to encourage and educate viewers. It was an all around interesting experience for me and my colleagues because we all learned from it.

The only restriction I was given after I had the surgery was not to rub my eyes for six months; I was so scared, I didn't rub them for years! Just kidding...but I really was cautious about rubbing my eyes for a long while. I had a series of checkups at certain milestones, like three months, six months and a year. I have had no setbacks at all...that's what happens when you don't rub your eyes! (Smiling)

Looking back, I was so glad to have my sight corrected. The most liberating thing about the surgery was that I was no longer that skinny four eyed kid. It was a morale booster for me. Having to wear glasses had created a kind of barrier between me and the rest of the world and now I am completely free and it has made a difference in how I feel about myself as well as in my appearance.

Advice to Readers

One thing I would say is that we see a lot of people these days having Botox, face lifts and plastic surgery and we have different reactions to it, some of them negative. I think that if there is any medical enhancement you can have that will improve your daily life and your outlook, it is worth whatever you have to pay for it. I always tell people that, man, when I get old, I am having it *all* done...the fat sucked out, hair regenerated, whatever. I am getting it all! It is worth it to invest in yourself, whatever it takes, because of what you are going to get out of it every single day. It will make you a more upbeat person to be around. You will be a more positive influence on others.

Having laser surgery is more than just not having to wear glasses anymore. It seems like a little procedure but it will change your life in ways you couldn't imagine. Being free of glasses is only a very small part of it. It's worth the investment in yourself for quality of life benefits it will bring you on a daily basis. My wife is actually starting to think about it and I have encouraged her with this same advice.

It takes a certain amount of courage to put the care of your eyes in the hands of someone else. The one thing that gave me the courage to do it was when I sat and talked to Dr. Price. He was so calm and that made me feel confidence in him. The person you choose should inspire you and make you feel confident. I have met some doctors that I wouldn't let wash my car! Some people you meet give you a positive reaction and then there are others you just have a bad feeling about. Trust your intuition.

I also didn't want a temporary solution that would wind up with me needing to go back in five years and have it fixed all over again. There are lots of ads out there and some of us think that all doctors are the same. They're not! Check around, talk to people and find a doctor you can trust. Look around at the facility, too; look and see if they have state of the art equipment. Are they staying on top of their game? Look at what certificates are on the wall, too; is this doctor someone

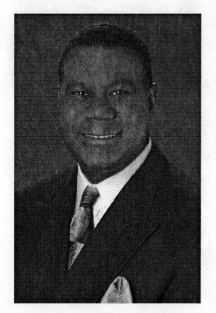

who is continually upgrading his knowledge and skills? It makes me very nervous when I see only one degree on the wall. That tells me that he went to school and now he's all done learning. I want someone who is invested in continually growing and learning to perfect his skills.

I am definitely glad I had laser surgery. It's been liberating!

Chris Wright

Other Conditions

I interviewed Linda Flinchum, joined by Lynnie, her husband, at the kitchen table of their beautiful home in Fishers, Indiana. Linda recalled how life suddenly changed one December morning in 2001 when she awoke to feel an odd weakness in her left eyelid that eventually worsened and led to blindness. Her husband's loving companionship and the care of a skilled, patient and persistent doctor she refers to as her "security blanket" strengthened her journey of faith and courage.

In the spring of 2000, I went for my annual eye exam with the intent of being fitted for bifocal contact lenses. My doctor agreed and worked with my eyes for the next six months, but the lenses just never fit right. They slid up and around in my eyes, and would not stay in place. Finally, I asked him to fit me with a pair of regular contact lenses, the same type I had worn for 40 years. Once I got those, I could see really well, so I didn't even bother to go back and have my eyes checked in September. There were no signs of coming trouble with my vision.

The Unexpected Happens

I was unprepared, therefore, for what happened on the first day of December. I got up as usual and started to rub my eyes the way I always did, but there was an odd sensation in my left eye. It felt like there were no muscles in my eyelid. I decided I better leave the lens out of that eye for a few days to see how I'd do. I never put it back in. My vision kept getting worse and worse, until all I could see was total whiteness. I went back to my optometrist, and he started me on several rounds of medication over the next two months, but nothing improved. Then in February 2001 he sent me to Dr. Price in Indianapolis for a consultation.

I felt a sense of urgency and was grateful when Dr. Price worked me in to be seen by Dr. Faye Peters the very next day. She took one look at my eye and quickly left the exam room to go get Dr. Price. He said my left eye was eighty- percent defective and I had a short procedure the next day to remove scar tissue that he thought might be the cause. I went back after 2-3 days with no improvement. Dr. Price also thought it might be herpes, and put me on medication to treat it. After a few weeks, he could see it was not doing me any good, however, so he took me off it.

Emotionally, I was having trouble coping; it had all happened so suddenly. I had some days when I went into the clinic crying. His staff was always so supportive and kind; they showed a lot of empathetic understanding. And Dr. Price was persistent and patient; he just would not give up. He was determined to help me, and he was always so positive and calm.

In April, he did an exploratory surgery and took tiny snips of tissue and sent them to a lab for biopsy and cultures. He ran so many tests that I don't remember all of them. The condition was hard to identify and even the lab had trouble figuring it out. The results came back and the mystery was solved: microscopic amoebas, called acanthamoebas, had gotten into a tiny rip in my cornea and had started multiplying. The more they multiplied, the blinder I became.

Dr. Price told me that most people with this condition are in extreme pain, but I was very lucky. I did not have any so I must have a pretty high threshold for pain. My eye ran a lot, though, and it was not very pretty to look at. I got into the habit of wearing dark sunglasses most of the time, even when going out to eat in restaurants.

The condition I had was unusual enough that very little research has ever been done, so there is not even a medicine to treat it. I was given a kind of bleach solution that was mixed at an apothecary and put into eye drops. I used the drops about ten times a day, a messy process to say the least.

When I first began seeing Dr. Price, I had appointments about two or three times a week. (Someone on the team counted them up and there were 110 visits!) I think he did this for two reasons: to see how I was progressing, and I think it was also his way of helping me get through it emotionally. He always reassured me at every appointment; he's a knee patter and he would tell me, "You're going to be okay" and then he'd pat me on the knee. When he was finally able to stretch my appointments out a bit more, I realized I had come to depend on him like a security blanket. Sometimes we'd pull into the parking lot and I would tell Lynnie, "Here we are at my home away from home."

The Transplant: A New Beginning

I understood that I might have to have a corneal transplant before it was all over. At some point, I told Dr. Price that I would like to save my own cornea, if we could. His exact words were, "You would certainly be better off with your own cornea." The eye drops destroyed some of the amoebas, but then they would develop immunity and start multiplying again. Finally, in May 2002, Dr. Price recommended and performed a corneal transplant in my left eye.

The procedure itself was not hard to get through; I just had to lie really still as he operated. I can remember overhearing Dr. Price saying that he'd been to his college reunion and how some of his classmates were getting ready to retire. He said he thought it was too early for that and I remember whispering to him, "Dr. Price you can't retire; I need you." He heard me and we both grinned and some of the nurses chuckled along with us. I suppose it is hard to imagine that you could have that kind of exchange during surgery, but it was a calm and comfortable atmosphere that Dr. Price created.

Ten months after surgery, he began taking out my stitches, and then in June 2003, he performed a relaxing incision. It was not a painful procedure, but I felt pressure on my eye during it and I was glad when it was over. A month later, I had cataract surgery to restore my vision in that eye even more fully.

Even though I had already been through a lot, four months later I also chose to have LASIK on that eye, too. This procedure is actually done in two stages and was well worth it because I just did not want to cope with glasses unless I absolutely had to. And by then I completely trusted Dr. Price, so I just marched right in there and had it done.

Occasionally I also developed tiny filaments that felt like scratches on my eyes, and I would have to go back to the clinic to get them removed (You can see where those 110 visits came from!) I was glad when Dr. Price recently said, "Let's leave well enough alone now." I was in complete agreement.

Looking Back

My first impressions of Dr. Price and his people were all positive and they remain so today. They are so professional yet they are really good at getting to know their patients and putting everyone at ease. Dr. Peters and Dr. Kelley are fantastic, too. Everyone on his team has made Lynnie and I feel like we are family, and I am especially grateful for Dr. Price's patience and persistence. He would not give up on me, and he reassured me of that each time that I saw him.

I learned an important lesson from this whole experience. I became blind without warning and it could happen to anyone. I certainly never expected it to happen to me but that was the challenge life gave me to face. It has given me a deep sense of appreciation for my eyesight and I will never take it for granted again. I enjoy my life and I enjoy being able to see the world I live in and the people I love. I am so grateful for everything that Dr. Price and his people did for me as I went through my ups and downs.

On a practical side, I have noticed that some of the more tedious things in life, like sewing, and reading, for example, take more concentration now. I have to pay more attention to details than before. I also think the whole experience has affected my nerves; it was such a long time going through all of it. I notice that I am uncomfortable driving in heavy traffic and some days I just feel more nervous overall, so I have had to adjust to these reactions.

As I have gotten older, I do think it's gotten easier to accept things so that has helped me adjust. My spiritual beliefs continue to bolster me, and I think you get back what you put into life. We both really like people and if I could name a guiding principle that I believe in, it would have to be the Golden Rule; that is what my husband and I both live by.

Advice to Readers

Don't be afraid; if there is something new that can help you, don't be afraid to try it. Your experience might also help someone else someday. I encourage you to take life one day at a time and be patient with yourself and listen to what your doctor tells you.

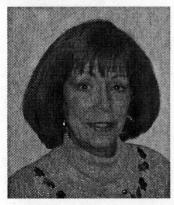

Linda Flinchum

Other Conditions

"A Healing Process"

Joe Young is a big man with a kind smile, a shock of white hair, and a deep voice bearing the trace of a New England accent although he's resided in Florida for many years. A devout Catholic, Joe's faith is what brings him courage and strength, along with his loving wife, Mary, and their family. A dreadful childhood accident left him blind in one eye until new hope was discovered in a casual conversation over dinner one night with Dr. and Mrs. Frank Price, Sr.

When I was fourteen a friend hit a marble with a baseball bat and I happened to be in the way. From that day on for the next fifty-one years, I was blind in my right eye and it was "frozen" (had no tracking movements). By the time I found Dr. Price, I had almost given up hope to ever be able to have my sight restored.

My family and I lived in Boston when the accident happened to me, and they took me to Mass Eye and Ear Hospital, one of the best medical facilities in the world. Doctors there did the best they could with the existing technology of that time. I had surgery several times and once I had to stay in the hospital for 30 days during which I was not allowed to turn over in bed. I had to lay still and be turned over by the nursing staff. Over the years, I had consultations with a series of doctors and not one of them gave me any words of encouragement.

Fortuitous Dinner Conversation

Fast forward fifty-one years and my wife and I were out to dinner with Dr. Frank Price, Sr. and I learned that his son, Dr. Francis W. Price, Jr., was a world-famous ophthalmologist. My wife and I talked it over that night when we returned home, and I called Dr. Price, Jr. the next morning. He asked for my medical records in order to study them. In a few days, we talked again and set an appointment. My wife, Mary, and I flew up to Indianapolis, and I recall it was a Monday morning when we met Dr. Price for the first time.

The thing that impressed us the most was how thorough and nice the people were on his staff. That plus the high-end technology and equipment they had was pretty amazing. They ran a bunch of tests and then Dr. Price came in and said "Let's schedule cataract surgery for Wednesday morning." My wife Mary and I spent a very restless night on that Tuesday night, as I recall. We had a lot of anticipation and it wasn't much fun, frankly, but we got through it.

Dr. Price told us beforehand that a normal cataract procedure would take about 15 minutes. He said he thought mine would take 30 minutes; on the morning when he began it took him two and a half-hours before he was done. He said it was one of the worst cataracts he'd ever seen. It was so hard that they had to use both manual efforts and ultrasound to break it up. About halfway through the procedure the anesthesiologist had to administer more medication to carry me through the remaining surgery.

Dr. Price removed the cataract, and he also stabilized my eye by inserting a capsular tension ring during surgery. It is used to increase the safety of cataract surgery in high-risk patients like me and the Foundation was part of a clinical study to see how well it worked. I was pleased to be part of the study and to help other people. That was a bonus beyond the opportunity to have the surgery to restore my sight.

The surgery required many stitches but it was painless. I was partially awake and could respond to Dr. Price's directions during the operation. He would remind me now and then to lay still and remain quiet as he worked. He, of course, was under the same restrictions because his work is so delicate and precise. He explained things to me as he worked and it was very reassuring to hear his voice. It made me feel calm.

Once I came out of the recovery room, Mary and I went back to our hotel that afternoon, I took a nap, and then we went out to dinner that night. We went back to see Dr. Price in the office the next day and two or three times during our stay. In the last visit he took the stitches out. My poor wife sat right there in the room with us and she couldn't look while he did it. It was harder on her than it was on me!

Vision Restored

As a result of the surgery, I regained peripheral vision, and my right eye moves naturally and "tracks" so it looks more normal. I don't have a cataract blocking my vision any longer and, while I cannot read, much of my daily life has been restored to me. I can see colors, for example, and it's just great.

A friend of mine, Jack Wagner, was going to have eye surgery awhile ago. I described the whole procedure to him, and encouraged him to relax as much as possible and not to worry. Not surprisingly, he had as good an experience with Dr. Price as I did. Over the years, I have sent about five or six people to Dr. Price because I have total confidence in him. It makes me feel good when people's lives are improved after their surgery. It's great to be a part of that healing process.

The greatest life lesson for me now that I have sight again is the sense of appreciation I feel being able to see colors and light. I never take it for granted and every day I feel very fortunate to have had this surgery. I get emotional when I talk about it because it changed my world so drastically and I am deeply grateful.

Advice to Readers

People are afraid to have anything done to their eyes and it's a natural fear. I think you have to just pull your bootstraps up, decide to do it, and have faith in your caregiver.

If anyone reading this book has any fear of eye surgery, you should know that if you are coming to see Dr. Price, he is so wonderful, so skilled, and so good at his work that there is no need for you to worry. You will be in good hands. I think of him as a miracle worker. I had been every place in the United States to get my eye worked on and no one would do anything until I met him. The end result has been great.

To readers who might not be able to reach Dr. Price, look for someone who has the same characteristics as he does: caring, highly skilled and experienced, and someone surrounded by an excellent team of professionals who treat you like you are family.

It amazes me that he is so talented yet he is also so down to earth; he and his wife, Marianne, are terrific people and wonderful parents.

I have to say a few words about his staff, too. They are really loyal and that's unusual these days; a lot of them have worked with him for many years. He is doing things right to make that happen. Let me share an example of what I mean about the kindness of his staff. A few years ago, I went to the Foundation's annual golf outing and I met a couple of the nurses and technicians that work for Dr. Price and they were so friendly to me. They each asked me how I was doing, and gave me a hug. I could feel that they really cared about how I had progressed since they had last seen me. It was an expression of their genuine and heartfelt interest in me and in my wife that touched us both.

I draw strength and courage from my faith, my dear wife Mary and my loving family. I have two wonderful kids, my son Andrew, and my daughter, Heather. In addition, I have two beautiful granddaughters, Madison and Mackenzie. We are a tight family and close to each other. Even though they live in the Boston area, we get together regularly. We are a Catholic family and our faith keeps us close. One of the best memories I have after surgery is when I went to church and really saw the inside of it for the first time. It was such a beautiful gift and I was filled with great joy. I am so grateful for these memories and for my life.

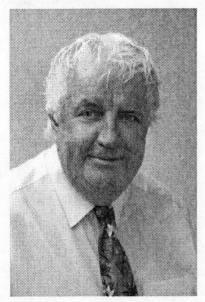

Joe Young

About the Cornea Research Foundation of America

More Americans than ever face the threat of blindness from age-related eye disease. The National Eye Institute estimates that over one million Americans aged 40 and over are currently blind and 2.4 million more are visually impaired. These numbers are expected to double over the next 40 years as the Baby Boomer generation ages.

Vision scientists at the Cornea Research Foundation of America (CRFA) in Indiana are pursuing world-class clinical research and physician/patient education to reverse the rising tide of blinding eye disorders. Our comprehensive databases and prolific publication of the latest innovations in ocular medical and surgical techniques offer a unique resource for ophthalmologist worldwide.

Our mission was established in 1988 by our founder, Dr. Francis Price, Jr., M.D., a respected entrepreneur with a passion for discovering new surgical techniques and treatments that sustain long-term visual recovery after corneal transplantation. His commitment to the preservation and restoration of vision is demonstrated by his status as having performed the largest number of small incision cornea transplants in the world. This new cornea-sparing transplant can help those with Fuch's dystrophy or endothelial dysfunction achieve a rapid visual recovery in 1-3 months without suture-related problems or difficulties with astigmatism.

Although not as commonly publicized as kidney or heart transplant surgery, corneal transplant surgery is the most widely performed transplant surgery today. More than 600,000 have been performed on patients who range in age from nine days to 107 years of age. Over 90% of all corneal transplants are successful in restoring vision.

The cornea is the clear front surface of the eye that can become clouded, distorted or scarred by injury, disease or hereditary defects. A condition termed keratoconus, a thinning of the cornea that can lead to severe nearsightedness or astigmatism, is one of the most common reasons for corneal transplants in North America. CRFA conducts studies to determine the cause of this and other vision-robbing conditions.

About 120 million Americans wear eyeglasses or contact lenses to correct the most common of all vision problems: nearsightedness, farsightedness or astigmatism. These are called refractive errors and affect the cornea. CRFA has participated in many multi-center studies and sponsored single site studies to develop more effective treatments in this area, including the use of corneal inserts to allow those over the age of 45 to regain reading vision.

How to Donate

The Foundation depends solely on donations from individuals, organizations and grants. Each year, we undertake at least 12 new corneal studies. The focus of many of the studies are in areas where there is little or no corporate or government funding - such as tracking corneal transplant results. And because it is not a medical school or a residency program, the Cornea Research Foundation of America does not qualify for most organized funding sources such as Research to Prevent Blindness. We depend on donations, therefore, for survival.

You give to make a difference in the lives of others. When people struggle to overcome an obstacle in their path, you help them. Your charitable gifts touch those in need today and your generosity builds solutions for the future.

Like you, the Foundation also touches the future. With your donation, we will continue to create your vision of a better world. Our work, and the lives it reaches, can be part of your legacy of love. We invite your partnership in making a difference.

To make a donation, please send your check to: The Cornea Research Foundation of America, 9002 North Meridian Street, Ste. 212, Indianapolis, IN. 46260.

The Cornea Research Foundation of America, Inc. is a 501 © 3 non-profit entity. Your gift is tax deductible to the full extent of the law. Federal ID # 31-1243592.

Thank you for helping us make a difference through research!

Glossary

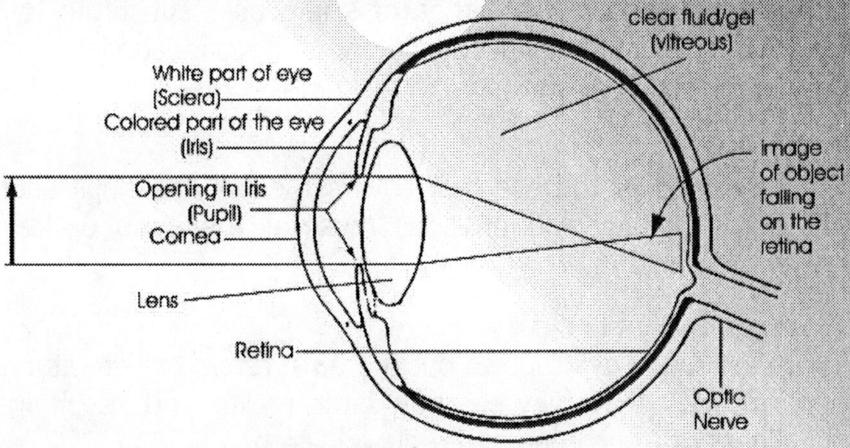
clear fluid/gel
(vitreous)
White part of eye
(Sclera)
Colored part of the eye
(Iris)
Opening in Iris
(Pupil)
Cornea
Lens
Retina
image
of object
falling
on the
retina
Optic
Nerve

CROSS SECTION OF THE EYE

Anterior Chamber

The fluid-filled space inside the eye between the iris and the innermost corneal surface, or endothelium.

Astigmatism

The cornea or lens is shaped like a spoon, causing light to focus on two points; symptoms are squinting and ghost images. Eyeglasses or contact lens corrects it.

Bullous Keratopathy

Small blister-like pockets ("bulli") form in the swollen corneal epithelial layer which greatly reduces vision (see also Fuchs' Dystrophy).

Cataract
Characterized by cloudiness of the crystalline lens that may prevent a clear image from forming on the retina. Surgical removal of the lens may be necessary if visual loss becomes significant. May be caused by damage, trauma, disease or aging or may be congenital.

Contact Lens
An optical device, consisting of small plastic discs with optical correction, worn on the cornea or sclera as a substitute for eyeglasses. Sometimes used as a protective bandage lens for an eye with corneal disease.

Cornea
The "window" of the eye that covers the iris, the pupil and anterior chamber, and provides most of the eye's optical power.

Corneal Dystrophy
There are many dystrophies but the term refers to hereditary abnormalities that may develop later in life and result in cloudiness of the cornea and reduced vision.

Corneal Graft, Corneal Transplant and/or Keratoplasty
Surgical procedure in which a scarred or diseased cornea is replaced with clear corneal tissue from a donor. (See also lamellar keratoplasty, penetrating keratoplasty)

Corneal Ulcer
Condition in which an area of corneal tissue is lost from the corneal surface. Usually caused by a fungal, bacterial or viral infection.

Descemet's Membrane
An anatomical term describing a thin, elastic layer deep in the cornea formed by the endothelium.

Endothelium
The innermost layer of cells in the cornea whose job it is to pump fluid, keeping the cornea clear.

Epithelium
The outer layer of cells in the eye which includes the cornea, conjunctiva and eyelid.

Far-sightedness or hyperopia
A refractive error in which light rays coming from a distant object strike the retina before coming into sharp focus. Usually corrected with eyeglasses or contact lens and sometimes by the eye itself as it accomodates to the condition.

Fuchs' Dystrophy
A hereditary condition that results in cloudiness characterized by guttata, epithelial blisters, reduced vision and pain. (See also Bullous keratopathy, and guttata.)

Glaucoma
Condition associated with increased intraocular pressure. If untreated, results in gradual, painless, irreversible loss of vision.

Guttata
Small, clear bumps on Descemet's membrane on the inner surface of the cornea. (See also Fuchs' Dystrophy)

Iris
An anatomical term referring to the colored tissue that lies behind the cornea and gives the eye its color as well as controls the amount of light that enters the eye, like the aperture, or F-stop, of a camera.

Keratoconus
A hereditary and degenerative corneal disease characterized by thinning and cone-shaped protrusion of the cornea. It usually affects both eyes and begins in the teens or early twenties.

Keratoplasty
Also known as a corneal transplant or a corneal graft; a surgical procedure in which a scarred or diseased cornea is replaced with a clear cornea from a donor.

Lamellar Keratoplasty or graft
Also known as a partial-thickness graft; a surgical procedure in which outer corneal layers are replaced with normal corneal tissue from a donor. (See also corneal transplant or penetrating keratoplasty)

Laser
An instrument that refers to "Light Amplification by Stimulated Emission of Radiation." It is used to purposely remove or separate tissues of the eye for various clinical purposes. There are many types of lasers, i.e. argon laser and yag laser.

Lens
The intraocular tissue that brings rays of light to focus on the retina; also an optical term referring to a piece of glass or transparent material used to focus light.

Myopia
A refractive error known as nearsightedness in which light rays from distant objects are brought to focus on the front of the retina. Without correction, individuals can see upclose but not far away.

Presbyopia
Also known as "old age vision," a refractive condition in which there is a diminished power of accommodation arising from the loss of elasticity of the lens that occurs with aging. Individuals cannot change focus from far away to upclose.

Pupil
The black circular opening in the center of the iris that regulates the amount of light that enters the eye.

Relaxing Incision

A surgical procedure in which linear cuts are used to reduce excessive tension in the tissue after corneal surgery, and reduce astigmatism.

20/20 Vision

"Normal" visual acuity. The first number refers to the patient's ability to see standarized symbols on a chart 20 feet away; the second indicates how many feet away a "normal" eye would see the same size symbols. If 20/40 vision, one sees at 20 feet what a "normal" eye sees 40 feet away.

Ulcer or Corneal Ulcer

Corneal tissues are inflamed, infected or lost and the condition is often associated with inflammatory cells in the cornea and anterior chamber. Usually caused by viral, fungal or bacterial infection.

Printed in the United States
49035LVS00004B/1-186